DUALITY

Founded by C. K. Ogden

The International Library of Psychology

INDIVIDUAL DIFFERENCES
In 21 Volumes

DUALITY

A Study in the Psycho-Analysis of Race

R N BRADLEY

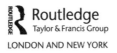

Routledge
Taylor & Francis Group
LONDON AND NEW YORK

First published in 1923 by
Routledge

Reprinted in 1999, 2001 by
Routledge
2 Park Square, Milton Park, Abingdon, Oxon, OX14 4RN

Simultaneously published in the USA and Canada by Routledge

711 Third Avenue, New York, NY 10017

Transferred to Digital Printing 2007

Routledge is an imprint of the Taylor & Francis Group

First issued in paperback 2013

British Library Cataloguing in Publication Data
A CIP catalogue record for this book
is available from the British Library

Duality

ISBN 978-0-415-21053-9 (hbk)
ISBN 978-0-415-86447-3 (pbk)

Our wills and fates do so contrary run

PREFACE

This book was originally intended as a sequel to *Malta and the Mediterranean Race,* wherein the prehistoric features of Malta are considered in the light of Sergian anthropology. When I returned to England from Malta I found that I had only touched on the fringe of the race question, which seemed more and more to permeate history, politics, and even human evolution. In its first shape the book was purely racial, and also fuller than it is now of ethnological detail. But the war came, and theoretical ethnology gave way to practical.

Yet the war proved the importance of the theme and, in a way, this book may indicate some of the deeper causes of that great conflict. For I have tried to shew that it was not an isolated event, but a culmination of a struggle pervading several millenia. Every age and every country seems at some period to experience its struggle of the long-heads and the short ; while in Ireland the conflict is eternal.

I have tried to shew how religion and politics are expressions of this strife, but it was only through the delay caused by the war that my eyes were opened to a larger and more important aspect of the question.

PREFACE

Being cut off from other literary activities, I turned to Freud and encompassed most of the Freudian literature. Then, caught for a while in spiritualistic current, I was led to Geley, Coué, and the French school of psychoanalysts. While Freud excels on the empiric side, the French, and particularly Geley, appear to possess more philosophic breadth. Geley seems to offer a magnificent philosophy of life, according well with the spirit which inspires both Bergson and Maeterlinck.

So many important and conflicting things have been said of late with regard to the conscious and unconscious, that it seems necessary to co-ordinate them in some measure, and this, in the psychological portion of my book, I have attempted to do. I have tried to envisage the wood as distinct from the trees.

I have treated of the conscious as something in the nature of a rebellion, but a rebellion which could be useful in the evolutionary sense. Most of the evils of the present day appear to be due to its hypertrophy. This is being generally recognised, and by none more clearly than Mr. Bertrand Russell, who is of opinion that we have been wasting our time. We have been thinking where we should have been seeing, and Professor Rutherford's recent experiments with the atom or the scientific treatises of Professor Eddington now reveal to us how much nearer to the truth the experimental method can bring us than can the idealistic. Our heads have been swollen almost to the closing of our eyes.

The significance of these psychological excursions for the purpose of this volume was that it revealed to me

PREFACE

that beyond the duality of race there existed a psychological duality ; and, more important, that they were the same duality. The long-heads were the unconscious race, the short-heads the conscious. The cleavage was of much the same nature as the sex cleavage, a division for higher development. The course of all is through strife to love, finality being reached in a true blend or marriage.

It may be thought that my division of the races into African and Asiatic may be too facile, but it is based on Sergi, who, like Freud, seems to possess an insight which penetrates beyond mere intellectualism ; and it does not appear to me that those who have tried to improve upon Sergi have arrived at any very tangible conclusions. In any case, wherever long and short-heads originated, they seem to be the same kind of long and shortheads, and that is sufficient for the purposes of this book.

As to the fixing of the races, most of my arguments are linguistic, and I have done no more than indicate them herein. I hope in course of time to publish the linguistic arguments in full. They support Sergi in an almost uncanny fashion, indicating two distinct language origins among Europeans, African and Asiatic. Our old " Aryan " or " Indo-European " languages turn out to be not Asiatic at all but, as far as vocabulary is concerned, pure Arabic, pointing back to an original Hamitic or African. So that the main body of the speakers must have been Mediterranean Race. On the fringes and sporadically we find the agglutination of the Altaic or Ugro-Finnic, which is Asiatic.

PREFACE

I have dealt somewhat fully with the literary aspects of " duality," the great exponent of which to-day is Mr. Galsworthy. The duality complex is one of the most important in literature. From this and other points of view many quotations have been introduced, and I hasten to express my thanks and make my acknowledgments for them. I have to thank Mr. Galsworthy and Messrs. Heinemann for permission to quote from *The Forsyte Saga ;* Mr. John Lane, of the Bodley Head, for quotations from H. S. Chamberlain's *Foundations of the Nineteenth Century ;* Mr. A. G. Tansley for quotations from *The New Psychology ;* Messrs. W. Collins Sons & Co. for quotations from Dr. Geley's *From the Unconscious to the Conscious ;* Mr. Havelock Ellis for quotations from *Man and Woman;* Messrs. Heinemann for quotation from Jacque Vontade's *The English Soul;* Messrs. Harper & Bros. of New York for quotations from O. Henry's *Options ;* Messrs. George Allen & Unwin for quotations from Maeterlinck's *Life of the Bee* and *Wisdom and Destiny ;* thanks are due to Professor Percy Gardner and Messrs. Macmillan for quotations from *The Principles of Greek Art ;* the extracts from *Susan Lenox, Her Fall and Rise*, by David Graham Phillips, are made by permission of the publishers, Messrs. D. Appleton and Co., of New York, the owners of the copyright. Finally, and not without sadness, I acknowledge my indebtedness to the late Dr. Sophie Bryant for quotations and most valuable material from *The Genius of the Gael*, one of the truest and most fascinating ethnological studies I know.

R. N. B.

Hampstead,
    December 1922

CONTENTS

CHAPTER I

SKULLS AND RACES

In Deniker's *Races of Man* will be found tables giving the measurements, not only of the skulls of all the human race, but of most parts of the body also. The reader need not fear that I am going to worry him with a mass of detail of this kind ; there will be too little rather than too much. Discussions on head-shape were at one time much in the foreground, but suddenly all interest seemed to cease, and that before any definite conclusions had been reached. The real reason was that all the theories were based on a false foundation and, when it was found that the old Aryans were not what we supposed they were, all the earlier arguments appeared to be discredited. Cranial theories culminated in the Franco-Prussian war, and the victory of the Prussians gave great prestige to the Aryanists with their hypothesis of an

Asiatic invasion of Europe in prehistoric times. Founded apparently on such vague statements that all light comes from the East, they grew in strength and detail until Ihering could tell us the exact time of the year at which the Aryans left their Asiatic home, and Houston Chamberlain was able to gather Christ into the Aryan fold. Chamberlain's *Foundations of the Nineteenth Century* is full of most interesting psychology, which is in fact more implicit than explicit. If anyone was a true Asiatic, that man is H. S. Chamberlain, and no one has ever understood or sympathized with the Asiatic mind as he has. I shall draw on him largely in the matter of racial psychology; the only trouble is that he has generally ascribed his characters to the wrong original peoples. His theory is that the Aryan or Asiatic skull is the long skull, and that was the view generally held in his day. This mistake was in great measure due to the discovery of the German Row-graves, in which the skulls were long. They seemed to belong to the oldest inhabitants of the land, and were adopted by the Germans as their ancestors. At the same time Max Müller was working out his system of Aryan languages of which Sanskrit, an Asiatic language, then appeared to be the most ancient.

A theoretical Aryan language seemed to require a theoretical Aryan people to speak it. The word Aryan was then supposed to mean *noble*, which fitted in very well with the traditions and aspirations of the Germans. Pieced together the Aryan theory amounted to this : Europe was in prehistoric times inhabited by a race of savages without culture or apparently any language until from the highlands of Central Asia there overflowed stream after stream of Aryans who endowed Europe with religion, light and culture. They brought us the language we speak, and we owe everything to them.

The theory became discredited largely on account of the discoveries of an ancient and advanced civilization in Crete, and this led people to turn to their Herodotus, full of facts, observation and local detail, and to discover that his supposed fabrications had far more truth in them than the theories and ideas beneath which they had been so long buried. His information aboute Crete was confirmed by recent discoveries, and attention was naturally turned to the Pelasgians, the indigenous peoples of ancient Athens, the Carians, Libyans, Iberians and Ligurians, all autochthonous peoples, and evidently of some account before the Hellenes

were heard of. It was then discovered that
Greek culture, especially that of Athens, owed
its essence not to Asiatic invaders, but to the
indigenous peoples, and that the Parthenon is
but a continuation of the culture which produced
the Palace of Minos.

The greatest illumination of the subject came
however from Professor Sergi at Rome, who in
his book *The Mediterranean Race* minutely
examines prehistoric skulls, and demonstrates
their origination. He is inclined to disregard
the old numerical measurements, which are
rather too precise for far-reaching ethnological
hypotheses. Broadly speaking, skulls belong to
two types, long and short; they are dolichocephalic or brachycephalic. The length of the
skull from the forehead to the back of the head
is compared with its breadth between the ears,
and the percentage of the breadth to the length
gives the cephalic index. If the breadth is 75
per cent. of the length or under, the skull is
dolichocephalic; if 80 or over, it is brachycephalic; between the two it is mesaticephalic.
But Sergi does not trouble much about these
numbers. There are two distinct kinds of skulls,
the long and the short, and skulls, being parts
of the body least liable to variation, are for him

the clearest indications of race. In neolithic times, which are significant for our present arrangements, Europe and a large part of Asia were densely populated by a long-headed people whom Sergi supposes to have originated in Africa. Although there may be some doubt as to the place of origin, I have my own reasons for assurance that Africa was their original home. These reasons are linguistic, and cannot adequately be dealt with here. These people are called by Sergi the Hamitic, Eurafrican, or Mediterranean Race. The remains of their megalithic structures are still to be seen throughout Europe, in Asia, Egypt and North Africa. They were the dolmen-builders, and constructed our Long Barrows. They embraced the ancient Cretans, the Ligurians, Pelasgians, Carians, Egyptians and Iberians, and are the substratum of European population to-day.

I do not propose to enter here into the question of their monuments and buildings ; to some extent I have done that already in *Malta and the Mediterranean Race ;* it is rather with their psychological aspect that I am concerned.

Their great flourishing period seems to have been about 3000 B.C., but by this time a new race was already making itself felt in Egypt, a short-

headed race, ultimately developing into the
pyramid-builders. It has been said that the
passport of these people into Europe was the use
of metals.

We have to think of a Europe thickly populated from Ireland to Russia and from Scandinavia to Sicily with long-headed men, with a
developed civilization and strong religious
tendencies embracing a worship of an Earth-
Mother who combined the qualities of Ge and
Aphrodite, and complicated rites bearing on love
and fertility ; their numerous sanctuaries tell us
that, in Crete, Malta, Ireland ; and Stonehenge
shews us that the invaders adopted and carried
on the ancient religion in a modified form.
The Asiatics did not come at first as an
invading and conquering horde ; they were not
by any means numerous ; their advance was
peaceful, their manners even servile. From
numerous sources we gather that they wormed
their way in, never letting the mailed fist be felt
until the gloved hand had done its work. They
dominated Sparta but never Athens, whose
aristocrats had ever the market-place to consider.
At Rome we see more precisely what happened.
Tarquin, still bearing his Mongolian name of
Tar Khan, the tribe chief, inveigled himself into

power, and his house incurred disaster through trying too soon to make that power hereditary. Neolithic Europe was matriarchal, power descending through the mother ; Tarquin attempted to institute father-right.

Matriarchy was evidently associated with polyandry ; a woman had whom she would for as long as she pleased, and Frazer tells us in *The Golden Bough* how these amorous and unfettered Mediterranean women were wont to take slaves as their mates. Modern women have asked me why, and the answer would probably be interesting. Possibly for the same reason as modern man has a *penchant* for barmaids. The dominant male always had his *hetairæ ;* the dominant female liked hers. It was an escape from the normal and conventional. There may be another reason also : it is woman's function to draw the race back to its origins, to average, to normalize ; for that reason she seeks to bring extremes within her net ; and the more the male diverges in his experimentalism, the more she seeks to acquire the benefits of such experiments for her offspring. It is in such a way that the race develops.

It is a trite saying that there is nothing new under the sun, and this is especially true in ethnology. What happens once happens again ; and what happens now has happened before. Have we no concrete example of the manner in which these Asiatics came to Europe ? Assuredly we have. As I shall shew later, they were a Mongoloid people, with dark lank hair, high cheek bones, yellowish complexions, with eyes set somewhat askew. Their ornaments were gaudy, bizarre and angular. They came wheedling, ingratiating, peddling their wares—the new metal implements. We think at once of the gipsies, of the travelling tinker, of Wayland Smith. Judging from their somatic characters no less than their language and habits, I feel convinced that the gipsies are but belated remnants of these old invaders.

Beneath their guile, however, they had qualities of blood and iron which in time gave them dominion over practically every country in Europe. Every nation of our continent seems to suffer at some time or other the domination of these hard and forceful men. From the Balkans they came down upon Greece as the Hellenes, and a later migration established the Dorians in Sparta and other strongholds of Asiatic culture. The invaders have many names, but they are essentially all one people, what is generally known as the *homo alpinus*, the true Celt. And it may be well at this point to clear up a misunderstanding as to what the Celt really is. Many people speak to-day of their Celtic qualities, to wit, emotion, spiritualism, second-sight, instinct, inclinations towards poetry and the arts. These qualities are not Celtic at all ; if you want to see the true Celt, you must turn to-day to the Prussian, practical, ruthless, bullet-headed man ; or Cromwell and his Ironsides. The mistake has arisen because the Celts were the advance-guards of the Asiatics in Europe, and were the first to be absorbed by a very absorbent race ; the method of peaceful penetration doubtless assisted. The Irishman, or the Highlander, who are popularly supposed to embody the Celtic qualities, are really pre-Celts, Mediterraneans. With the Lowland Scot it is a different matter ; he is an Angle, a true Celt, and an Asiatic.

In prehistoric times these Celts overflowed across the Alps as Oscans, Umbrians and Sabines. The last became the patricians at Rome, the plebeians being the old Ligurian population. The higher classes in the Roman army are associated with the horse and the round shield, both Asiatic ; the lower classes bore the long

shield of the Mediterraneans.   And it may be
observed here that the symbol of the Asiatics is
roundness, and of the Hamites or Mediterraneans,
length : long head, long barrow, long shield ;
round head, round barrow, round shield ; the
difference is vital and permeates both character
and culture.

In the same way Western Europe was gradu-
ally dominated by successive hordes, Gaels,
Brythons, Teutons ; and at various times came
the less diluted Finns, Lapps, Magyars, Huns and
Turks.   The more diluted they are, the more
normal their features ; the purer, the more
Mongolian.   The purest retain some form of
Mongolian language.

It is interesting to consider the nature of our
own domination.   Owing to our great racial
admixture it may be thought difficult to isolate
this particular phenomenon.   Our first historic
Asiatic invaders were the Goidels or Gaels, who,
although very much mixed with the indigenous
population, must still to some extent be reckoned
as belonging to the invading horde.   They
appear to be almost uniformly long-headed and
are now little distinguishable from the Mediterraneans.   The Brythones or Britons, however,
who, as the Ordovices, split the Welsh in twain,
seem to me, in spite of surmises to the contrary,

to have been more definitely short-headed, and it is probably from them that so many Welshmen inherit the short head. The next invaders of our islands, Angles, Saxons and Jutes are similarly divided. Professor Ridgeway tells us in *The Early Age of Greece* that the Angles cremated their dead, while the Saxons and Jutes probably buried theirs. This distinction in funeral customs is found also in Rome, where the older families clung to indigenous custom of burial, and is vital. Mediterraneans buried, Asiatics burned. Not only by this primitive custom are Angles and Saxons divided, but also by their head-shapes and their characters. The Saxon, owing to admixture, has a long head and a long face; his manners are genial and easy; his character gentle and inclined to be slothful. East Anglia on the other hand is the home of dissent, methodists, quakers, hard-headed, dour business-men; of Cromwell, his Ironsides and his cavalry; they take pride in their horses. It is said that the East Anglian fisherman follows the fish, while the Devonian waits for the fish to come to him. Among the East Anglians the Roman nose is still seen, and sometimes Mongolian features. It is a land of stern housefathers.

Similar characters are found in the Anglian lowlanders of Scotland, Puritanism, character, logic, mathematics, philosophy, sternness, justice, pure intellectualism.

When the Angles of England and Scotland joined together under Cromwell against the Stuarts with their Cavaliers and Catholic tendencies, we suffered our first real Roundhead domination. It is no co-incidence that these people were called *Roundheads* at the time, for unconsciously races, especially when in close contact with their rivals, are inclined to emphasize somatic distinctions. In the South of France women artificially lengthen the skulls of their children in the cradle ; the Laze around Batum shorten their children's skulls. And the distinction is often emphasized by dress and toilet. The Northern Italians, the Prussians and the Danes wear their hair *en brosse* to emphasize the shortness of their heads. Our street Arabs are wont to plaster their hair down over their foreheads to add an apparent length to the head. Artists, Bohemians and other Mediterraneans wear their hair long, and I shall always remember taking a Scotch friend to a vegetarian restaurant in Soho, frequented by actors and artists, and his first remark : " Some of these people want their hair cut." The racial significance of the flowing locks of the Cavaliers, and the close crop of the Roundheads, in this manner becomes clear.

Instances of these peculiarities in dress could be multiplied indefinitely, but I might say a word on moustaches and whiskers. The Mongol could grow a poor sort of bristly moustache, but no beard, whence in our army, an Asiatic institution, moustaches are favoured, but not beards ; an exception was made, however, when, during the war, traditions were broken down, and men of the other race were brought in. In the Navy, which is Mediterranean, one must be clean-shaven or wear a full set.

Cromwellian traditions, embracing Puritanism, the Scotch Sabbath, system, progress, empire, whiggery, the Bank of England, five per cent, friendliness with Germany and suspicion of France, lasted until the death of Queen Victoria, the accession of Edward VII., and the *entente*, when we threw off Puritanism as a garment, ranged ourselves on the side of the Mediterranean Powers against Germany, and indulged in colour, dancing and Bohemianism generally. The Great War in which the Mediterraneans joined together against the Central Powers or Asiatics marks a definite reversion to Mediterraneanism ; nor is this to be wondered at in the

light of Ripley's *Races of Europe*.   Here we see
the Asiatics, the *homo Alpinus*, inserting themselves as a wedge along the mountains of Europe.
Like a glacier they glide down and cover Europe
to its furthest extremities.   Then gradually the
glaciation recedes towards its mountains; Greece,
Italy, Scandinavia, and finally Britain are uncovered, and the old long-headed race is left
somatically much as it was before.   What is the
broader significance of these events ?   We may
get some inlking in the following chapters.

CHAPTER II

THE SIGNIFICANCE OF SKULLS

I

I have sketched in brief outline the history of the skull question and indicated its altered aspect. It is not wise, however, to be too dogmatic concerning origins which are necessarily obscured by the lapse of so many centuries. In *Man, Past and Present*, Professor Keane thinks that Sergi has erred on the side of simplicity and, whilst admitting the African and Asiatic homes of the long and short-heads respectively, argues for a second and earlier round-headed race from Africa. That, prior to the coming of the Mediterraneans, there were short-headed men in Europe, I am only too ready to admit, for some of the pre-Mediterranean types show the effects of short-headed crossing, but I am doubtful about the early brachycephals coming from Africa. In Irish and even in Welsh there seem to me to be traces of the agglutinative speech of the Asiatics, and it is very possible that in some localities the Mediterraneans found broad-headed predecessors, but I think they were still Asiatics.

When *Malta and the Mediterranean Race* was published I was surprised to find considerable opposition to the suggestion that there could be any link between ourselves and the ancient Mediterraneans. That such a relationship exists and is acknowledged by our foremost archæologists, the following quotation from Professor Elliot Smith's *Ancient Egyptians* will shew : " So striking is the family likeness between the early neolithic peoples of the British Isles and the Mediterranean and the bulk of the population, both ancient and modern, of Egypt and East Africa, that the description of the bones of an early Briton of that remote epoch might apply in all essential details to an inhabitant of Somaliland."

Of course there must be modifications of the theory ; things did not happen altogether as Sergi suspected. He thought that the Hamites crossed from Africa by the Straits of Gibraltar, Malta and Sicily, and the Greek Islands ; but I feel convinced on linguistic grounds that such was not the case. I cannot enter into the argument here, for it is both elaborate and contentious ; nor is it very significant for present purposes. Suffice it to say that I have become more and more convinced that the Hamites, dwelling in North Africa, passed through Egypt, where they founded the Egyptian civilization, thence to Arabia and Syria, to Asia Minor, whence they spread over Europe. Both language and Greek mythology support this view.

Another question which arises is this : why start from neolithic man ? In discussion I find that inquirers ask about the pithecanthropus, Neanderthal, Rhodesian, Piltdown and Cro-Magnon man. These do not as a matter of fact very much affect the question of modern civilization. The first four, with their low foreheads, prominent brow-ridges and heavy chinless jaws, are some of Nature's experiments in mankind, tried, found unsatisfactory, and left by the wayside. Sporadically, even in modern times, they crop up, and one at least attained a bishopric. Cro-Magnon man was on a different footing, and is regarded by some as one of the finest types ever evolved. Lofty in stature, with a long, high head, he had a Mongolian cast of features, shewing that even in these early days there was still a race blending of the same kind as we find to-day. It is not improbable that he still persists, and I think I have on occasions met him. But one of the most ancient and persistent types is the normal long-headed man such as you meet in London to-day; Sir Arthur Keith thinks he goes back to palæolithic and river-drift days. We must remember, however, that the northern part of Europe was subject in early days to glaciation and man went back and fore with the ice-sheet. With palæolithic man there is a gap in culture if not entirely in race, and our development takes a new start in neolithic man.

Whatever may have been the population of Europe in neolithic days the coming of the Eurafricans, or Mediterraneans, is so clearly indicated by monuments, notably the dolmen-stream, and language, that we must admit that with their coming there was something in the nature of a new beginning.

2

I have spoken much of long heads and short, and shewn how the measurement is taken. Sergi, ignoring indices, finds that each type of skull falls into different shapes, as viewed from above: among the dolichocephals we have the ovoid, pentagonoid, elliptical and so forth ; and among the brachycephals the beloid, sphenoid and others. These terms are valuable in practical work, and I have found them extremely useful in examining skulls, both ancient and modern. But to the merely interested, these distinctions are useless for ordinary observation purposes. I am writing from the point of view of living psychology and propose to deal with the types as we meet them in the street.

From this point of view it is very convenient that the shape of the face usually follows that of the head. Long-headed man has a long face, and *vice versa*. There are the inevitable exceptions, disharmonic types such as are found in Austria, with short heads and long faces. But the general rule will suffice for our ordinary faces. Great Britain has in the main reverted to the long-headed type, and that is the kind you generally meet. The other type is met occasionally, and is the easier to exemplify in that he is the dominant, successful man, who is often portrayed in the newspapers. I might instance Sir Eric Geddes, Mr. Shortt, Lord Kitchener, Lord Beatty, and, for earlier times, Cromwell and Mendel. Professor Elliot Smith has drawn attention to traits other than the short head ; for instance, the long ramus of the jaw, giving the square chin of our men of action ; and the oblique eye-socket, relic of Mongolism. Those who care to examine the skulls in the Pitt-Rivers collection at Oxford will observe that the eye-socket is not so much oblique as square, and squarely set. But it is manifestly different from the oval eye-socket of the Mediterraneans, the outer and upper corners of which are not so high. This abnormal setting of the eyes leads to a characteristic feature of the short-heads, their bad sight. Most short-headed men wear spectacles and in Germany the fact is notorious ; but this defect is compensated for, to mention only one character, by excellent teeth. While the Mediterranean is a seer, the Asiatic is a biter as well as a thinker.

Types of long-headed men are more common, and amongst them we might cite as examples the Prince of Wales and his brothers, the Bishop of London and Lord Lascelles.

When it is evident that these ancient racial types are the ordinary people we meet, it will perhaps be recognized that skull-shapes have an importance which should not be suffered to lapse into obscurity. It may be wondered perhaps why I should rake up a question which was thought to be dead. But if it has died as a question, it is always with us in our politics and our life, in how many and in what subtle ways I intend to shew. I have said that prominence to the question was given by the first Franco-Prussian war, and the question now takes the first order of importance with the second Franco-Prussian, or Great World War. I have referred to the fact that this was a combination of the Mediterraneans against the Central or "Asiatic" Powers, of the long-heads against the short. It has been recognized as a *Kultur*-war, a war of contending cultures and civilizations. As I pursue my theme I shall try to shew what was the essence of those civilizations, the inner core of the peoples' psychology.

Nor is the Great War an isolated instance of the struggle ; it seems to be one of the essential conflicts of mankind. In the Great War we had on the one side short-heads, Asiatics, system, co-ordination, intellect, logic, philosophy, will, direct action, the mailed fist, Puritanism, male domination, big battalions, the land army ; on the other, long-heads, Mediterraneans, art, poetry, impulse, instinct, emotion, invention, a growing feminism, colonies, sea-power. We have seen these combinations before : Athens against Sparta in the Peloponnesian War ; the North and the South in America ; Puritans and Roundheads in our own country ; to give but a few examples.

The question has not only a historical importance ; we live in the days of a new psychology, a new evolution. This seemingly eternal duality in human history is paralleled in psychology by those two great aspects of mentality now brought into prominence by the Freudians. It will be observed from the characters I have given that one race in some degree represents the conscious, and the other the unconscious, and I shall shew that it is more than a question of mere similarity. This cleavage of the race into two warring factions, this similar cleavage of the mind into conscious and unconscious, leads us to a further cleavage, the great and obvious cleavage of nature, sex. As I proceed it will be seen that the sex duality has no little in common with the others, and later, when we come to consider the new light thrown on evolution by Geley, Maeterlinck and Bergson, that nature appears to proceed by this duality as if unity and finality could only eventuate by way of cleavage and opposition ; and the argument will be strengthened by reference to recent discoveries as to the nature of electricity.

3

Some years ago when I had studied only the
racial aspect of the question, I had the pleasant,
if unusual, experience of staying with an
Anglican Father exiled in the heart of Crom-
wellism. I was surprised at the permanence of
the old spirit of the Roundheads. It was near
St. Ives, in Huntingdon, and the atmosphere was,
I was surprised to find, still full of the historical
feeling. The situation afforded me a curious
object lesson. The Father was a remarkable
man, of Irish birth, and thoroughly Irish in his
nature ; Irish of the best kind. Coloured prints
of St. Columba hung on the walls of his poor but
beautiful dwelling, and he himself seemed
inspired with that form of Christianity which
claims to be as old as Rome, as it is independent
thereof. Ascetically trained, he rose early every
day to toll the bell of his church, of which he
was often both priest and congregation ; service
over, he returned to perform the most menial
duties of the household. It was part of his life
of service. His face was lean, but its lines were
noble, and his grey eyes had the most humorous
sparkle. His tales were the most rollicking,
mainly curious experiences of his own. On
festive occasions he brewed an admirable punch,

and then jests sparkled with the wine. Amid
the dull rolling plough-land he had created for
himself out of an old school-house bungalow and
its plot of land a beautiful oasis, with a wind-
screen of poplars planted by himself.

He was a real Irishman and prided himself on
being known to the police, for, as an ardent
socialist, he had taken part in riotous meetings
in Trafalgar Square. All this fits in very well
with Ireland but not with the Church of England,
and banishment to this most uncongenial spot
in England was his punishment. Of course the
dour East Anglicans regarded his every word
and action with suspicion, and his High Church
ritual found little favour with these sombre
dissenters. Once when he was benighted on a
strange road a trap overtook him. He was
granted a lift, but rather as a matter of duty
than otherwise. " We Methody," said the
farmer, " we no Bigamy," which being inter-
preted meant that if they were Methodists they
were not bigoted.

He did what he could to get into touch with
the young people of the place, and thought this
could best be done by telling them some of his
more youthful escapades. He told them how he
went into a bank and, finding a dour dissenter

there waiting for the cashier, he suggested that his companion should keep watch while he jumped over the counter and seized the money. The point of the tale was, however, entirely missed by the audience. "How much did you get, father?" inquired one of the lads, and the father's reputation was not enhanced. Rather was he regarded as an emissary of the devil and a representative of the Scarlet Woman.

I told him how the position fitted into my racial views, and he was enormously interested. And one day, when I had been dwelling on the permanence of the struggle, he asked me if it was to go on for ever, or whether some solution could not be found in the end. According to my lights I answered that I thought it would always be so. He took me more seriously than I had taken myself, and to my astonishment spent a sleepless night. But reflection brought him consolation in a text—"Seek ye out the old paths." I did not see how this applied and nor did I press him on the point; I was only too glad he had found comfort. I wonder still what this text meant to him, but later, when I thought of it, it seemed to me rather apposite. Sir Arthur Evans shortly afterwards gave a lecture on Ancient Egypt—how the newest fashions were

really the oldest. We have seen this illustrated
in Ancient Crete, where the women wore low
necks and flounced petticoats, corseting themselves severely. Their coiffures were Parisian,
and the ladies would not have been out of place
in our ball-rooms. The Spartans, Romans,
Puritans and Quakers did not tolerate these
sexual advertisements and clothed their women
as far as possible in straight lines so that sexual
distinctions should be obliterated. But *naturam
expellas furca*, woman will always be woman, and
to-day she revels in her rediscovered Mediterraneanism. There is something very apposite in
Eothen : " You know what a sad and sombre
decorum it is that outwardly reigns through the
lands oppressed by Moslem sway. The Mahommedans make beauty their prisoner, and enforce
such a stern and gloomy morality, or at all
events such a frightfully close resemblance of
it, that far and long the weary traveller may go
without catching one glimpse of outward happiness. By a strange chance in these latter days,
it happened that, alone of all the places in the
land, this Bethlehem, the native village of
our Lord, escaped the moral yoke of the
Mussulman, and heard again, after ages of
dull oppression, the cheering clatter of social

freedom, and the voices of laughing girls."

For Mahommedans you may substitute Spartans, Turks, Prussians, Puritans or Lowlanders; they are all Asiatics, but with their individual differences.

I do not think the father thought of this, or perhaps he only felt it unconsciously. He may have been thinking of his Irish Catholicism in which the new is bound ever to the old so that new and old are one. But the incident set me thinking, for one could not leave the world perpetually struggling, a prey to accidental faction. Mr. Bradley, in *Appearance and Reality*, suggests that we may be taking an unwarrantable liberty in speaking of inorganic matter; we do so merely because we cannot see the organism; but the organism may yet exist. In the same way I am less and less inclined to regard things as casual, and when this conflict appeared so permanent the more it seemed to require a purpose. Such a purpose seems strangely enough to have been sensed in a way by the ancients themselves, but it seems to have become more clear through recent researches in psychology.

CHAPTER III

CHARACTERS OF THE RACES

I

It must not be supposed that any long-headed or short-headed man you meet will necessarily possess a definitely long-headed or short-headed character. There are mixtures and disguises, and also a transcendentalism of character rising above race. Some fall in with the traditions and feelings of their herd ; others react violently against their environment and become the opposite of their real nature.

Mr. H. G. Wells refers in another connexion to *pseudomorphs*, wolves as it were in sheep's clothing, or *vice versa*, and the word is rather significant for our purpose. We sometimes meet men who are somatically of one type and psychologically of another. But whereas you occasionally find long-heads with short-headed characters, especially in Scotland, the reverse is in my experience seldom found.

In this connexion one naturally thinks of the Mendelian characters of dominance and recessiveness ; which of the two races is the dominant ? We have observed in the short-headed peoples a definite charcater of political dominance, but this is not quite the same thing as hereditary dominance. An aspect of the subject was studied by Dr. Beddoe in a Vienna lying-in hospital, and he found that a broad-headed child had more difficulty in birth than a long-headed ; he came to the conclusion that nature favours the dolichocephals. The reason for this is that in the ordinary course of nature the shape of a child's head bears a definite relation to that of its mother's pelvis. Long-headed mothers have a pelvis which is so shaped that a long-headed child can pass through it. The child's head, so large in proportion to its body, is always the critical factor in birth but, given purity of race there is, at least in primitive times, little difficulty. But with the invasion of the short-heads there arose some serious complications. The male sex preponderated among them, and when conflicts with the indigenous peoples came, the males of the latter would be slain or made prisoners, and the females would naturally be seized by the conquerors. The new generation would have long-headed mothers and short-headed fathers, and, as it is extremely difficult for a broad head to pass through a disharmonic pelvis, the dice were loaded against them. In a mixed population like Austria it was probably this problem which confronted Dr. Beddoe.

This aspect is purely mechanical, and has perhaps little relation to hereditary dominance. Historically, however, it is observed that one of the most conspicuous features of the Mediterranean Race is their power of absorption. Where to-day are the short-headed dominants of ancient Greece and Rome ? Where are our own short-heads or those of Scandinavia ? Professor Ripley shews that in these countries there has been an almost complete reversion. In Irish history it has always been an acknowledged fact that any wanderers outside the Pale were promptly absorbed in race and character by the Irishry. The fact is that the Mediterranean Race is like woman ; she is there first and last ; she suffers male domination for her own purposes ; she accepts the male, particularly of the aberrant type, that she may absorb his qualities into the race ; but like woman the long-headed race is eternal. It concedes an accidental dominance that it may conserve the essential.

It is in this connexion that the question of pseudomorphism gains some importance, for, if by degrees the short-head everywhere disappears before the long, one wonders whether any benefit has been gained by the racial clash. It seems to me that in these pseudomorphs lies our main hope of saving any definite good from the conflict.

After indicating that character does not always necessarily follow somatic features, it will be interesting to consider how far the parallelism exists, and this is best accomplished by considering isolated peoples in their essentials. It may be difficult to single out the qualities of an Englishman, but even this is not difficult of accomplishment by a Frenchman or Italian, whose culture is essentially different from our own. It is necessary to separate the accidental from the essential, the transcendental from the natural; and by first studying more primitive and unmixed peoples we shall be able to trace essential racial characters through modern peoples. That there are definite long-headed and short-headed characters is indisputable, and I shall attempt to shew later that such characters have a broad significance in the evolutionary scheme. We will now proceed briefly to isolate as far as possible these racial characters.

2

In Babylon there was once a mixture of foreigners; the legend of the tower of Babel typifies the clash of Semite and Akkadian, the African and the Asiatic. The culture of the latter made Babylon's greatness. The Babylonians were gifted with practical common-sense and considerable forcefulness of character. They introduced bricks and rectangular architecture. Abandoning the naturalistic method of numeration used by the Mediterraneans, the decimal system of the ten fingers, they invented the duodecimal, permitting of division by 2, 3, 4 and 6. They also invented the Sabbath—so dear to Asiatics—not for religious purposes, but in order to get more work out of their employees.

The Hittites, known to us from the Bible, were a confederation of tribes, and Garstang, in his *Land of the Hittites*, shews that they were mixed, embracing both long and short-headed elements. The Mongolian element, however, is very distinct; they wear pigtails and shew the well-known facial characteristics. They spoke Mongolian, their language being related to Etruscan, Turkish and Akkadian. Among them we find an original mother-worship which becomes overlaid with that of a father-god. A meeting in procession of the male and female deities is shewn in the rock sculptures of Iasily Kaya, and Garstang thinks that this meeting is intended to induce fertility. This may well be the case, but it is not impossible that the meeting of the gods signifies a blending of the races both for fertility and stability. In character the Hittites were mediocre, but of great vitality. They were a settled people, cultivators; practical and genial; keen traders and cunning.

This stability of character is found also among the Bigoudens, the mongoloid people of Pont l'Abbé in Brittany. In *Vagabond Days in Brittany*, Mr. Richardson describes them thus: they are ugly, with high prominent cheek-bones and flat noses; their hair is lank and very black. They love finery, wearing gaudy clothes, embroidery and gold lace. They are industrious and practical, full of quiet energy; Pont l'Abbé is no backwater. Some significance attaches to their ornaments, which are of a garish nature, reminiscent of the Hittite and Turkish, even the Russian, and favouring the geometrical.

Our authority for the character of the Mongols is Jeremiah Curtin (*The Mongols*). Rooseveldt speaks of their anonymous victories. They were

the introducers of the bureaucracy of the Chinese
pattern, so much favoured in Europe, and it is
to this spirit we owe our competitive examina-
tions for the Civil Service. The Mongolians had
a childish reverence for learning. They were
accomplished women-snatchers, women being
regarded as chattels. Great hunters, hawkers
and riders, they were also great eaters and
drinkers. They were characterized by love of
power, and followed tangible, material objects.
Temudjin is noted for his ruthless singleness of
aim, his instinct for power and for self-preserva-
tion. They set great store on the spoken word,
regarding oaths and promises as sacred. Like
the Spartans, they boasted that they were not
traffickers or traders. They had the instinct of
alliance and of empire. The relations between
father and son and master and servant were of
great importance. Their slaves were thanes and
companions. Temudjin appointed his lords
marchers, his stewards, chamberlains, and officers
of the household. They were strong in cavalry
and had their lancer regiments. They made
sacrifices of maidens and horses, had a multitude
of wives, whose purity they guarded well.
Temudjin, afterwards Jenghiz Khan, killed over
eighteen million people in China and its neigh-

bourhood alone ; his last words were " Firm and
unbending is he who keeps a plighted word
faithfully," reminding us of Edward I.'s " Keep
troth." The Mongolian type of chivalry, their
stewards, cupbearers and the like have much in
common with feudal England. Their cavalry
are a link with the Roman patricians and our
Cromwellians. Their love of conquest and power,
and methods of obtaining them, remind us of the
Prussians.

In ancient Rome the Patricians were Sabines,
the plebs Ligurians—short-heads and long-heads
respectively (Ridgeway, *Who Were the Romans*).
We find a constant struggle between the two,
ending in many concessions to the plebs and to
the *jus gentium*. The Roman Empire and the
Roman Law are, however, short-headed institutions. The latter bristles with male dominance,
persisting to our own day. It specializes on
purity of race and wedding-cake marriage.
Ihering says they were a born nation of lawyers.
H. S. Chamberlain's view of them is very
interesting, as he has, so to speak, inside information (*Foundations of the Nineteenth Century*). He
says that the state and law were inseparable.
The upper ten thousand could only be soldiers
and lawyers ; the tradition, a little widened to

include the navy, church and diplomacy, was carried into Germany and England. Their greatness was anonymous. " In the case of the Roman tree everything went to wood." " The poet and the philosopher could not prosper in this atmosphere." The Roman was the first to regulate marriage. " His will extended even beyond death by the unconditional freedom of bequest, and the sanctity of the last testament." They " were the greatest masters in the abstraction of firm principles from the experience of life." They possessed " qualities of self-control, of abstraction, and the finest analysis."

The character of the Prussians has been manifested in the war, although it was pretty well known before. The authoress of *Elizabeth and Her German Garden* is very amusing in her references to the " man of wrath," and her *Caravaners* very happily brings out the male dominance. The Germans have always been noted for their idealism, basing the external world on their own views about it. The migratory ego, infusing an external object with its own complexion, flourished among them. Owing to this egostical kind of idealism they became quite out of touch with the feelings of others, cutting down, as it were, through the links of the unconscious. They lacked what Dr. Sophie Bryant calls other-consciousness, and so they were bad diplomatists. Idealism does not necessarily lead to philosophizing ; for philosophy is a product of repression. Expressed in singleness of aim and purpose it may lead to direct and forceful action, as we know it did. Moreover their intellectual type of mind perfected an excellent organization. Schopenhauer has said that " the real national characteristic of the Germans is dull-wittedness." We might almost say the same about the Scotch, both being slow, as it were, in the uptake. This quality, however, does not proceed from a lack of intellect but from its abundance. The short-heads are essentially intellectual, but intellect has its limitations. It creates a world of its own, cutting itself adrift from its environment. The more intellectual a man is, generally the more slow-witted he will appear to the man in the street, but his failure lies on the emotional and intuitive side. He has to construct every proposition consciously, receiving nothing as a concrete whole.

This analytical discussion of national character is apt to lead to misunderstanding, and for that reason I hasten to give the assurance that one shape of head is no better than another, and that if certain short-heads find themselves with strange bedfellows, it is Nature's fault and not mine. Both heads, both characters, have in them good and bad ; but what is more important is that they are essential ; they are the complements of each other, like male and female, conscious and unconscious. Each character bears within itself the germ of its nemesis ; as with the Cretans, who were liars, the Greeks ever at each other's throats, the Roman father unbending to excess, the Spartans or Mongols exceeding in cruelty, the Prussians in ruthless action. These qualities were given for moderate use, and it is their hypertrophy, while valuable for the purpose of scientific example, which is blameworthy.

The Lowland Scot must not therefore object to coming under review in this section, since the English are not altogether excluded ; for, whatever the shape of our heads, our culture is, or has been since Cromwell's time, of the short-headed type.

The Southern Scot is noted for his practicalness, his appreciation of money, his sureness and steadiness, and for his intellectuality. He is supposed not to be able to see a joke, and that is because he takes it too literally. He builds up

intellectually, but a joke often has a lacuna somewhere, and the Scot falls through the gap in the
ladder. Moreover it presupposes a kind of
emotional rapprochement between hearer and
speaker, which the Scotchman often lacks. The
main characteristics of the Lowlander are intellectualism and practicalness.

A very fascinating study of English character
is given by Jacque Vontade in *The English Soul*.
Coming from a Frenchwoman it naturally
emphasizes the non-Latin differences,—we may
say, the Asiatic elements of English character.
We are a mixed people, originally long-headed
and, after a period of short-headed domination,
reverting to dolichocephaly. Our culture is
largely that of the dominant short-heads.

The writer speaks of our " ever-present attitude of spiritual discipline," and the more I see
of France and the Latin peoples, the more this
expression appeals to me. The Englishman
loves discipline, not external, but self-imposed.
It is seen in his long walks, his cold baths, his
camping-out, the rigours of hunting, shooting
and fishing. The Mediterraneans can never
understand an Englishwoman walking when she
could take a cab—besides, it spoils the legs.
But, whatever an Englishman's weakness, he has

somewhere his particular form of discipline, overt or concealed.

She senses an Eastern relationship particularly in our manifestation of the will—" perhaps the civilization of the Orient has existed only to produce England." Comparing the Eton boy with Aladdin, she considers him " the triumph of the English will." " The Englishman wills with his invincible muscles." The will, discipline, exercise, are of course Roman characters, ultimately Asiatic, and it is interesting to note how naturally we have adopted the Roman mantle.

The Englishman hates superstition and Catholicism because he has no fear of God, who is a junior partner rather than a master; here we find the patriarchal tradition of the Hebrews. Death is also obnoxious to him; the Forsytes do not recognize it. Solidarity with the dead is a Mediterranean character; with the Mediterranean death is but a different kind of life; there is no real separation to-day and never has been. But the English get their dead out of the way as quickly as possible; the true Asiatic burned them, that no trace might remain. It is an essential difference between Protestantism and Catholicism.

" The English are unsurpassed hopers ";

this quality has some relation to their will-power and muscularity. They are often able to make their hopes come true. Mere hope, however, I do not regard as an essential Asiatic quality ; it is rather a form of the wish, the libido ; but there is all the difference between the successful and the unsuccessful hope.

Touching on sport she says : " Many of the very principles that created Imperial Rome, many of the dominating exclusive ideas of ancient Judea, are still fresh and operative in modern England."

One could expand these ideas to great length, but it is perhaps sufficient to note the appreciation of will-power, of patriarchal ideas, Protestantism, and sport. Vegetarianism and things of that kind are referred to an ascetism of the mind, harking back to the *exercitus* of Rome. Possibly cleanliness and sanitation are in part due to the same cause.

There is a charming story of the station master of Maidenhead, and his calmness and honesty with regard to the writer's furniture. This only illustrates the calm practicalness of the English. My French friends tell me we are so *pratique*. I think we may claim this character without discussion. The Englishman is usually calm and collected, that is, he is dominated by his conscious. They also tell me that we are kind to women and children ; it seems to me there is all the difference between the continental politeness, mere reaction to circumstances, and real kindness which belongs to the ideal content of the mind. Moreover through the world the Englishman has a reputation for honesty, reliability and character.

Of course he had numerous drawbacks, but the French lady kindly draws a veil over them.

3

The character of the long-heads is more elusive, for character is a speciality of the short-heads. We are almost reminded of Pope's saying with regard to women, that they have no character at all. But, if they have little character, the Mediterraneans have a very definite psychology. We are well aware of this from our acquaintance with the Latin nations, and our Mediterranean experiences.

Of course it is difficult to find the long-headed character undiluted in a nation, for there has been much admixture. We can only do what Jacque Vontade did for the English, specialize on differences. The French are racially mixed

as we are.   But the cultures are different, ours
being largely Asiatic, theirs Mediterranean.   The
long-heads of France live in the valleys and
towns, and it is they who count.

We can only infer the character of the early
Cretans.   St. Paul tells us that they were liars,
and we can easily believe it.   Regard for truth
and the spoken word is an Asiatic quality.   From
Mosso's various works, now somewhat eclipsed
by Sir Arthur Evans' scientific volume on the
Palace of Minos, we gather that they were
feminist, sexual and inclined to be socialistic.
Like the Kabyles and the early Irish, or even the
Greeks, they suffered from parochialism, and
burned each other's cities.   There was no
welding idea of unity—a lack of control.   This
same lack of control seemed at first to be shewn
in the arrangement of their buildings—magnificent structures, yet lacking the unity of those of
Periclean Athens ; from Sir Arthur Evans' work
we become more aware of a controlling Asiatic
element.   We gather. however, that their culture
was highly æsthetic and sensuous.

The Greeks were mixed, but the two races have
their culminations at various points—notably
Athens and Sparta.   The Peloponnesian war
was like our Great War, a conflict of races and

cultures—the Blue Water School, colonies, democracy and the Market Place against the Big Battalions, land power and militarism. The Athenian women wore grass-hoppers in their hair to shew that they were Pelasgians, or original Mediterraneans, and Greek culture is best typified by Athens. H. S. Chamberlain tells us (*Foundations of the Nineteenth Century*) that they were great for their poetry and art, and not for statesmanship, philosophy or bravery. They were not great metaphysicians. The Hindus are metaphysical, but the Greeks are great for their plastic power. They excelled in science, poetry, creative power and empiricism, but spoilt their work, says Chamberlain, by trying to explain transcendental work empirically. He condemns them, as he condemns Goethe, because of their clear sight and their sensuousness, for he naturally preferred the purely metaphysical and abstract mind of the Asiatics. If the real national characteristics of the German is dull-wittedness, that of the Athenians is assuredly the reverse. They had all their senses about them, and were keenly alert. They lived externally, not internally like the Asiatics, and responded freely to external stimuli. They were imbued with *joie de vivre* and lived fully in the present.

Touching their art, Professor Percy Gardner (*The Principles of Greek Art*) says that " the puritanism of the Dorians curbs the Ionian levity." The same difference crops up in contrasting Cretan and Greek architecture. Of course even the Athenians were mixed, but the Asiatic conscious and control were just sufficient to translate the emotion artistically without stifling it, as happened in Hittite or later Egyptian work. Thus " the Greek temple could only have arisen among a race in which the senses were extremely acute and active and the mind of a very clear and logical order." The wonderful proportions of their buildings arise from the " acuteness of the Greek senses." The beauty of their monuments is due to clearness of perception and taste.

The writer tells us that Dorian sculpture was athletic and military while the Ionian was decorative and soft. In poetry Homer and Hesiod represent the Ionic spirit, joyous freedom of life, curiosity, observation and powers of enjoyment.

He harps on the logic and bright intellectualism of Greek art, but this is different from logic and intellectualism of the Chamberlain type. In the one case the intellect is a means to an end and no more ; in the other it is intellect *per se*, with no external relations. He speaks of the beautiful relation of part to part ; that is, there is just enough conscious and control to make the product perfect. The conscious is subsidiary to the unconscious creative force.

We are told that Greek artists and writers aimed at effect ; they always had the audience in view ; they were other-conscious, like the Irishman or the Italian ; external.

The Ionic dress was folded and clinging ; the Dorian fell perpendicularly, swatching the body. The Mediterraneans, full of libido, were dominated by sex, and concealed it in the old days as little as the Parisienne does to-day. The Puritan Asiatic has always set his face against such expressions of the libido, and attempted to subdue sex. While the Asiatics did away entirely with their dead, with the Mediterraneans they were and are ever-present. The catacombs are reminiscent of prehistoric hypogaea or homes of the dead as still seen in Malta. There is reason to suppose that in prehistoric times living and dead remained beneath the same roof. Feast-tombs were common in Greece, and Solon passed a sumptuary law with regard to them. None who behold the grave-yard services in modern Italy on All Souls' Eve can deny the solidarity of this people with the dead, a truly Mediterranean feature. It is an aspect of the unconscious binding the present and the past, and has a close relation with the ancestor worship and idolatrous tendency of the long-heads. Religion was not a thing aloof, but a friendly association with external objects and perceived relations. To the Greek any bush or stream might represent a deity, and his religion, if more than skin-deep, was not much deeper than his senses.

We need not resort to history for an example of the continuing racial struggle. Some peoples have it soon, some late, some have it now. To-day it is the Irish question. The real Irish are true Mediterraneans ; Ulster means Lowland Scot, Presbyterian, prosperity, the covenanting spirit of the Scots and the Jews. Some say it is a religious struggle, but that only means that it is an ultimate racial conflict. The Irish are known to be of the Mediterranean Race and they are Catholic. The Presbyterians of Ulster are Angles from the Lowlands of Scotland, Cromwellians, or English dominants. The degree of their dissent marks the strength of Asiatic blood, of the *conscious* race.

But it is the true Irish character we want to analyse now, and that is sympathetically portrayed in Dr. Sophie Bryant's *Genius of the Gael.*

She tells of the absorbing power of the Irishry. They are conservative in ideas and primitive in instincts. They have " a less-developed instinct for pure negative self-control than any other people." Positive, irrepressible, original, full of personality, swift-willed, with wide intuitive grasp, they possess concrete minds, which react as a whole. Though the writer does not hint at it, we are reminded of the concrete imagination of Keats, the most typical of poets.

With them there is " a high degree of liability in the subconscious to pass into the conscious." " Inferior in the Teuton's gift of dogged executive " they have yet a " facility of consciousness." As a gloss we may say that their unconscious, unlike that of the Asiatics, is near the surface and easily emerges.

Their concreteness of mind makes for positiveness. As they are never under the dominance of one mood for long, lunacy and suicide are rare with them. This is an important point psychologically and is one of the advantages of what the psychologists call the *unstable* character.

While the Germans are—or were—the sentimentalists of Europe, the Irish have " the Celtic gift of accurate imaginative sympathy," " a miraculous insight into your wants." Here we must be warned that the " Celt " is not the ethnological Celt who is the same as the Teuton, but really the pre-Celt. As Dr. Bryant remarks, " the Celtic Gael has absorbed the Iberian."

" Fanaticism," continues the writer, " is near him." "An Irish crowd mobilizes with strange swiftness, and Irish politicians can co-operate unexpectedly with a rapidity embarassing to governments." They have intuitive social insight.

They excel in the *Aufschwung* sports, such as the high and long jump, and putting the hammer, rather than in the co-ordinative games, such as golf. Their games are merely the working off of the libido, and are characterized by swiftness and force.

Imbued with honour and knightly faith, family ties mean much to them. There is no desire for divorce. There are indeed *mariages de con-venance*, but they are successful owing to the equality of the sexes. Such equality is a feature of ancient Egypt, where the marriages were of a contractual nature. More truly it is a relic of the ancient dominance of women, a mother-right, which lingered so long on the fringes of the Roman Empire and was not entirely subdued in Sparta.

For the Irish Dr. Bryant coins the word *other-conscious*, significant both racially and psychologically. Other-consciousness is one of the conspicuous features of the Mediterraneans—a kind of solidarity with your neighbour, your environment, with past and future; sympathy and intuition; the birthright of the unconscious mind.

Truth, we are told, is not placed in Ireland upon so lofty a pedestal as with the Asiatics. The Mediterranean is inclined merely to respond to his environment, and there is lacking in him not only the control of the Asiatic, but possibly a moral idealism which finds more fruitful soil in the conscious mind. But there is a certain distinction about the Irish lying : " The Celt lies from excess of tact, the Saxon from defect of care." That is to say, both lie, but the Irishman, like the Cretan, is the more pleasant and natural liar. He responds to his environment and is inclined to say what you want him to say, or what the exigencies of the moment demand.

The Irishman's idealism is of a practical nature, like the Frenchman's. When solitary he becomes eccentric, but his mobility on the whole makes for stability, for it is corrected by social instinct. In the light of the newer psychology, one might venture to suggest a further explanation. It is the monomaniacs, the people with fixed ideas, who go mad, but if one sways backwards and forwards from one idea to another the swinging of the pendulum makes for sanity. One extreme corrects the other and reaction cancels action. Hence the Irishman's mobility makes for stability of a kind, at least it prevents eccentricity.

In politics, and here the writer is speaking of some years ago before the passions were stirred to their depths, Irish views are influenced by universal friendliness combined with conservative affection. The tribal idea remains, and Liberalism is softened by reverence. We have an example of the unconscious running into the future, but never cut off from the past; it is in fact external.

The Irish, we are told, are always primitive, and this character belongs to the essential femininity of the Mediterranean peoples. Stronger on the emotional than on the intellectual side, their literary genius is apt to exceed their mental powers. But true art is essentially unintellectual, the function of the conscious being merely regulative. For sheer beauty and direct feeling I think it is difficult to match Synge's *Shadow of the Glen*, as acted by Irish players.

There is, however, mental facility and a concrete unity of consciousness, the simple logic and architectonics which we observed among the Greeks.

Finally, as if to clinch their Mediterraneanism, Dr. Bryant remarks on their " social solidarity with the dead."

CHAPTER IV

RACIAL DIFFERENCES TO-DAY

I

Having isolated to some extent the characters of one or two races, it will be interesting if we pursue these racial distinctions into religion, politics, the workings of everyday life. The characters are so permanent, so essential, so complementary, that it is impossible to regard them as of fortuitous origin. They have a meaning in evolution, and may in a way be regarded as examples of an eternal duality.

Religion is perhaps of the greatest significance in this respect. A friend of mine recently remarked that if ever he took to religion—which was improbable—he would become a Quaker, or a Roman Catholic. These seem to represent the two extremes, the one relying on faith, the other abundant in works—the unconscious and the conscious.

The psychological view of religion is that it is non-moral, a primitive emotion. Statistics have been drawn up shewing even that its appeal is greatest to the immoral. The statistics are French, and refer to the Catholic Church. The English generally dissent from these views, for, being strongly Protestant, they specialize on ethics rather than religion. The Quakers are the strongest ethicists. But the English, even those who are purely ethical, like to think themselves religious. Being highly idealistic, they alter facts but like to regard them as unchanged.

Historically speaking, religion consists in faith, ceremonies, emotional exercises and the like. Its primitive forms are seen in Saturnalia, Bacchic dances, and corroborees. It has nothing whatever to do with goodness.

To the Englishman religion has everything to do with goodness ; that is, it has given place to ethics. If we persist in calling this religion we falsify both history and psychology. We may go to the mountain, but it is wrong to say that the mountain has come to us.

Religion is a natural emotional manifestation, belonging to man's unconscious life. When he begins deliberately to think of others, to sacrifice himself, to consider the interests of the community, he has broken with the pure unconscious. By thinking of others and denying himself he has brought that ideal content into his environment which we have seen belongs to the conscious. He has acquired the wisdom of which Maeterlinck writes : he has become detached, and has his own standards.

The Quakers are an interesting example not only because of their good works, but also on account of their association with East Anglia. Short-headed man was always a dissenter, and, wherever you find these people strongly developed, Wales, Kent, Hampshire, you find the countryside studded with their bethels. Protestantism is an embracing form of dissent, and is the essential religion of the Asiatics.

The Mediterranean people were matriarchal, and to them woman was not only the ancestor, but the priest and the god. In the Maltese sanctuaries numerous effigies are found representing an enormously developed woman, who to them typified both Gē, the earth mother, and Astarte or Venus. Their temples were abodes of love, and a tradition still clings to some of the Irish dolmens that if a maid meet a man there she can deny him nothing that he asks. Love and fertility were the essentials of the Mediterranean religion and the tradition still persists. The earth-mother and the goddess of love have been merged in the Virgin, but in Malta there is still considerable confusion. The Virgin is Stella Maris. And with us the church is still the abode of love and fertility, but it is a different kind of love. The love of God is insisted upon, but the church in country districts remains the natural meeting place of the sexes, and Church parade after the evening service at Worcester Cathedral is regulated by the police, not unaware of the workings of the Freudian unconscious, to such an extent that people walking one way must walk on one pavement, and those walking the other on the opposite. A woman does not feel properly married unless she is married in church, her unconscious harking back to primitive times.

But apart from these more material considerations there is a definite Catholic spirit which belongs to the Mediterraneans. Catholic means universal and the word bears unconscious testimony to that solidarity which binds together living and dead, past and future, man with his neighbours and surrounding nature. In this way the Irishman's liberalism is tempered by reverence. Mr. Calderon in criticising Tchekof

says that he deals with group emotions; the
question will be dealt with more fully when we
come to literature, but the group-tendency is
both Catholic and Mediterranean.

But we have not even yet reached the kernel of
Catholicism regarded in its opposition to Protestantism. It may be summed up in a very brief
phrase—the Protestant is above God and the
Catholic below Him. This is the secret of the
Greek *anagke* or necessity complex. The Greeks
felt that fate was too much for them; Jacque
Vontade would tell you that it is never too much
for the English. The Hebrews, strongly tinged
with Asiaticism, made covenants with their God;
he was an arbitrary, fickle, petty tyrant just as
they were. If he did not keep his part of the
bargain, no more would they. These Covenanters
have been perpetuated in both Scotland and
Ireland. From Jacque Vontade or Edmund
Gosse we can hear much of this god in the
cupboard, this private god; and " this old god
of ours " was as well known to the Kaiser as
to John Knox.

The English chaplain goes into the field as a
soldier and the Salvationist fights the devil in
full regimentals; but the French *padre* goes into
battle in cassock and soutane. There is no

swash-buckling with God. The Catholic's attitude is of humble submission.

2

"The Romans," says H. S. Chamberlain,
"quite insignificant in philosophy, were perfect
masters in the abstraction of firm principles from
the experience of life—a mastery which becomes
specially remarkable when we compare other
nations with them, as, for example, the
Athenians." I would lay the emphasis on
abstraction, an Asiatic characteristic; the
Mediterraneans were concrete. That is another
difference between Protestantism and Catholicism. The former owes its origin to various
Alpines, Luther, Calvin, Zwingli. Luther prided
himself on going straight to the fountain-head,
cutting out all intermediaries. Whereas the
Catholic requires sensuous aids, windows, vestments, statues, images, incense, the Protestant
is a sworn enemy of these material channels.
Cromwell and his Puritans specialized in icono-
clasm; the Presbyterians made the church into
a barn; the Quakers are guided by the inner
light.

The Mediterranean is a materialist, the Asiatic
an idealist.

It has sometimes seemed to me that, by a

curious formal extension, the one pursues the ideal
through the material, the other the material
through the ideal. It is so, but it may be only
accidental. For instance, the Catholic seems to
seek God, but always through the material;
the French are obviously keen bargainers, but
for the good of posterity or *la belle France*;
women also pursue the essentials, but in the
interests of their offspring and the eternal.
Whereas, if you judge by results, you find that
your idealist is generally none the worse off for
his idealism. The short-head is naturally
acquisitive. The two most idealistic nations are
probably the English and the Germans. Though
never lacking a moral pretext we seem to have
annexed a fair portion of the globe; and the
Germans have not been backward, at least in
their efforts.

A quotation from *Susan Lenox* bears on the
point :

" It is impossible for anyone, however stupid,
to stop long in Paris without beginning to idealize
the material side of life—for the French who
build solidly, first idealize food, clothing, shelter,
before going on to take up the higher side of
life—as a sane man builds his foundation before
his first storey, and so on, putting the observation

tower on last of all, instead of making an ass of himself trying to hang his tower to the stars. Our idealization goes forward haltingly and hypocritically because we try to build from the stars down, instead of from the ground up."

Idealism has its nemesis; it becomes the fashion to adopt its cloak, but with many it is merely a cloak, and you have the hypocrite and the humbug. Of course both types may fail from the point of view of absolute morality, if there is such a thing; but they fail in a different manner. This is well brought out in the *Price of Love* by Mr. Arnold Bennett. Louis Fores is a soft Mediterranean from the South of England. He wants to cut a dash; he lives for externals. There is something Italian in his nature. As he does not care for work, he steals; he is a common sneak thief. But he does not profess to be anything else. His cousin Julian Maldon is a dour Midlander, an Angle; a thief too, but with a difference. He steals from egotism, his confession is an apotheosis, in making it he towers above us. His idealism swamps the theft as a base detail. We often see this in England, especially among the more puritanical section. The idea, the principle is wonderful; the act is criminal. The phenomenon is often referred to as the migratory ego, and instances of it dominate German philosophy. The short-heads were eminently egotists, and the ego, though physically limited, is ideally unfettered. Externals do not worry it. An external object may be black, but if the ego sees white, it transfers whiteness to the object. Any form of subjection is hateful to it ; it scorns to be the product of nature and evolution. Finally idealistic philosophy asserts that all nature exists solely as an aspect of the ego. It maintains that the ego created its creator.

The Quakers are an extreme instance in that they represent a kind of transcendentalism. Coming of a warlike, dominant, acquisitive stock, they more than any others seem to have beaten their swords into ploughshares. Their abstraction, their subservience to the inner light, are Asiatic qualities ; but, in that they have thrown off the cumbrous formalities of their religion and become our most significant ethicists, they represent an aspect of the conscious which will be further considered as we look more closely into its nature.

Ethics are transcendental, but religion is natural. If in its essence it is an emotion, in its form it is racial, as in Ireland to-day. Religious ceremonies are manifestations of corporate race feelings and traditions. In our politics we have the same racial conflict ; we have two parties because we are composed of two races, but in politics the more psychological race differences are emphasized. The tradition runs from Cromwell and the Roundheads through the Whigs to the Liberals on the one hand, and from the Cavaliers through the Tories to the Conservatives on the other. The one party is characterized by Dissent, cocoa and intellect, the other by orthodoxy, beer and emotion. It is apparent therefore that pure race features are transcended and that here we rise into the psychological realms of the conscious and the unconscious. The question may be elaborated at a later stage, but for the moment we will leave it.

Numerous other aspects might be mentioned ; in art, the naturalism of the Mediterranean and the conventionalism of the Asiatic ; in education, the theoreticalness of Froebel and the sense-impressionism of Montessori ; in philosophy the idealism of the orthodox and the evolutionism of Heraclitus, Bergson and Maeterlinck. The duality is all-pervading, but it is always in some degree the same duality, and we must content ourselves with certain aspects.

CHAPTER V

DUALITY IN LITERATURE

The contrast of English and Irish is a favourite topic with our dramatists and novelists, especially at the present moment. "Peg o' my Heart," "Paddy the Next Best Thing," "Salad Days," are but three instances testifying to English interest in racial contrast. The last-mentioned novel hardly aspires to first rank in literature, but is perhaps on that account the more interesting, in that Mr. Burke slams in his effects with greater *naïveté*. There are no nuances in the drawl, affectation, control, reserve, studied mannerism, self-consciousness of Dick, nor in the unrestrained emotionalism, impulsiveness, inconsequence, directness and simplicity of Judy. She has no complexes, he is full of them; the heavy control of his conscious manufactures them. Moreover the salient racial characteristics

in thought and morality are effectively if somewhat crudely thrust into the picture. Judy com-
ments on the fact that there are no divorces in
Ireland. Dick and his uncle, both men of
experience, are obsessed by sex—so much so that
they are on tenterhooks lest their skeleton
should peep out of the cupboard. To Judy and
the twins there is no sex problem ; it is all plain
sailing. The Irish girl, like the Frenchwoman,
can talk about it with startling openness, because
it has never been repressed. It is pure and free.

No book or play of this type is complete
without a satire on the Englishman's monocle,
" that bit of glass in your eye," as Paddy calls
it in the play. Few would suspect any real
racial significance in this trifling feature. But
like so many tricks of the dress and hair the
custom carries on a racial tradition. The
Mediterraneans pride themselves on their vision.
The Asiatics, marred by the myopia of the
mongoloid eye, find their compensation in brain-
power and metaphysics. The monocle, even if it
has no use, is still sometimes worn as a fashion,
in other words, as a racial distinction ; and
Martin Ross' shortsightedness was considered
a mark of aristocracy, that is, of alien blood, by
the Irish peasantry.

The contrast between English and Irish is popular in literature not solely for purely racial reasons ; rather because in concrete form it expresses essential distinctions, which may shew themselves in race, culture, sex or psychology. It is this contrast which makes a work eternal and significant, whether the author realises it or not. Generally it is only felt subconsciously, and no one perhaps sensed it more strongly though subconsciously than Goethe. It was perhaps more clearly realized by Schiller, a true Asiatic, although he did not and could not measure its full significance. Schiller is a good moral poet, but, as he candidly admits, lacking in natural magic. It is eternally to his credit that he realizes this so fully. One of his short philosophic essays, *On Naive and Sentimental Poetry*, distinguishes very clearly between the inevitable magic of a Goethe and his own laborious efforts ; and he harps upon the distinction in his correspondence with his friend. Sentimental poetry, as he calls it, is artificial, and deliberately constructed ; it has that " high seriousness " demanded by the great Victorian, Matthew Arnold ; it is static, analytical ; it passes through the hemispheres of the brain ; in a word, it is *conscious*. It is of the more classic character,

lacking that romantic fervour, which works
  " As effortless as woodland nooks
    Send violets up and paint them blue."
The magic of the word, the power of the flash,
the touch of colour, the more imponderable
qualities of the emotion, are strangers to Schiller,
as they are the birthright of Goethe. Wordsworth had more than an inkling of the vital
distinction.   Poetry should be " simple, sensuous,
passionate "—that is unconscious, Hamitic.
" Poetry is the spontaneous overflow of powerful
feelings " ; then, realizing that this is insufficient,
he adds, " it takes its origin from emotion
recollected in tranquillity." The last words give
the Asiatic touch. The recollection in tranquillity allows the emotion to pass through the
hemispheres of the brain, the conscious ; the
process gives Asiatic idealism and classic control.
Poetry must be licensed by the " censor," and
the censor was strong in Wordsworth's day.
We know that Coleridge escaped him by taking
opium, and sank into the limitless dreamland of
the unconscious. Wordsworth is inclined to fall
into extremes, the victim of an infantile unconscious, or a tyrannic conscious. But only a real
poet could write such a line as
  " Murmuring from Glaramara's inmost caves."

Goethe was not only fully aware of race conflict, he realized that he was its child.

" Vom Vater hab' ich die Statur,
    Des Lebens ernstes Führen ;
    Vom Mütterchen die Frohnatur
    Und Lust zu fabulieren,"

which is as much as to say that his father was an Asiatic and his mother a Hamite. Johann Goethe, the father, was a man of sterling integrity, esteeming himself and his position, tenacious of purpose, formal, pedagogic ; he might have hailed from the Lowlands of Scotland ; methodical, precise, a pillar of municipal life, steadfast as a rock before the buffets of fortune. Rebuilding his house from the top downward ; not artistic, but a patron of art ; a typical Baillie of a Scotch town. Stern of temper, even tyrannical, his autocracy was tempered by justice.

Goethe's mother, Frau Aja, as her friends called her, was something very different ; a bright and dainty creature, who could neither spell nor write straight. Her nature was poetic and artistic, and from her Goethe drew his love of telling stories. *Joie de vivre* she gave him, and the love of dressing up in startling finery when that wave of Hamitism, the *Sturm und*

Drang, swept over Germany ; the fondness for the society of actors. From her he drew that *Sehnsucht,* dissatisfaction with the present, craving for the distant, the past and the impossible ; longing for the sake of longing ; and the mysticism which she got from her own father. (M. Reeks, *The Mother of Goethe.*)

If he had been her child alone, we might have had but a poor, vapouring, *Sturm und Drang* youth, following the vagaries of mood, the urge of passion—a waster. But though he felt this within him, and could give rein to it in his poems, he yet felt the controlling nature of his father's character ; he was always aware of the censor :

" Wer groszes will, musz sich zusammenraffen,
In der Beschränkung zeigt sich erst der Meister,
Und das Gesetz nur kann uns Freiheit geben."

He realised the necessity of that rebirth through the conscious, the quelling and the mastering of " the terrible mother," and so the conscious and the unconscious go hand in hand, *Dichtung und Wahrheit, Natur und Kunst.* He was not only a poet of eternity, but also an able administrator and a man of science.

" Edel sei der Mensch,
Hilfreich und gut."

But the fairy gift was his mother's and, as

Frau Aja's biographer writes, " If the exterior is dominated by Herr Goethe's character, the interior will ever be loved for Frau Aja's sake."

The conflict of his ancestry forms a complex which he is constantly striving to dissipate in his works.   It crops up continually in his poems, and *Werther* and *Tasso* are among its expressions.

This complex is as widespread as it is enduring. Perhaps least of all should we expect to find it in America, but it is almost as strong there as in Europe.   A famous economist ascribed the American Civil War to economic causes ; others say the same of the Great War.   But these causes are not final.   It is said that the North waged war because they could not compete with slave labour, and there is some truth in this.   It is something remoter than the " small spark," the pretext of the conflict, but it is not final. When English industry migrated to the coal-fields, Sussex and Gloucestershire did not declare war on Lancashire and Stafford.   There is all the difference between the rivalry of a near relative and that of a stranger.

The Northern States of America were colonized by Puritan or Asiatic stock ; the southern by Cavalier or Mediterranean.   Probably O. Henry knew nothing about the more ultimate race

F

divisions, but he senses the sharp distinction. This will be observed in the story of *Thimble, Thimble*, in *Options*.

It is of two branches of the Carteret family, the founders of which both came to America in 1620, but in different ways—one as a Pilgrim Father, the other in his own brigantine, which landed him on the Virginia coast. " John became distinguished for piety and shrewdness in business ; Blandford for his pride, juleps, marksmanship and vast slave-cultivated plantations."

The Yankee Carterets went into the Leather Belting business in New York, a musty, arrogant and solid affair. It heard rumours of the Civil War, yet not enough to disturb the routine. But the war cost Blandford Carteret everything, including his life. So it came to pass that Blandford Carteret the Fifth, aged fifteen, was invited to come North and join the business, and at the age of twenty-five he sat equal partner with John, the Fifth, of the old firm.

Here the story begins. Old Uncle Jake had been entrusted to hand to the Virginia Carteret an ancient watch, a precious heirloom. He had not seen his young master for years, and both youths were just alike. They decided to play a joke on the old man, by giving no indication of

their identity and letting the old negro discover it.
The Northern youth said to his cousin :

" Bland, I've always had a consuming curiosity
to understand the difference that you haughty
Southerners believe to exist between " you all "
and the people of the North. Of course, I know
that you consider yourselves made out of finer
clay and look upon Adam as only a collateral
branch of your ancestry, but I don't know why.
I never could understand the difference between
us."—Blandford suggests that it lies in just
what his cousin does'nt understand.

So old Jake is called in to see if he can distin-
guish the alleged aristocratic superiority of the
" reb." He is of course utterly fogged by the
likeness, and determines to use strategy. But
neither young man gives himself away in answer
to the negro's questions, while he is determined
that the precious heirloom shall not fall into the
wrong hands.

" And then, to old Jake's relief, there came a
sudden distraction. Drama knocked at the
door with imperious knuckles, and forced Comedy
to the wings, and Drama peeped with smiling
but set face over the footlights."

Drama rustled in under the guise of a variety
star, Miss de Ormond. Black-tie conducts the

case, but blue-tie is evidently the defendant.
There is something about a rash promise of
marriage given after a wild night, and some one
is deeply involved. There is more than the
promise; there are letters. Their price is ten
thousand dollars, or the fulfilment of the engage-
ment to marry. Black-tie has been so far con-
ducting the case on thoroughly businesslike and
matter-of-fact lines. But Blue-tie is not going
to let his cousin do all the talking.

"I think it is time," interrupted Blue-tie,
"for me to be allowed to say a word or two.
You and I, cousin, belong to a family that has
held its head pretty high. You have been
brought up in a section of the country very
different from the one where our branch of the
family lived. Yet both of us are Carterets, even
if some of our ways and theories differ. You
remember, it is a tradition of the family, that no
Carteret ever failed in chivalry to a lady or failed
to keep his word when it was given."

"Then Blue-tie, with frank decision showing
on his countenance, turned to Miss de Ormond.

"Olivia," said he, "on what date will you
marry me?"

Before she could answer, Black-tie again
interposed.

He proceeds in his masterly fashion. "Chivalry is one of our words that changes its meaning every day. Family pride is a thing of many constructions—it may shew itself by maintaining a moth-eaten arrogance in a cobwebbed colonial mansion or by the prompt paying of one's debts."

The sharp rasp of a cheque torn from its book concludes the little scene, and the man of property emerges triumphant. "I've heard," says the lady in leaving, "that one of you was a Southerner—I wonder which one of you it is?" But no such doubt now obsessed Uncle Jake. "Young master," he said, "take yo' watch."

Of course the cultured reader would have given it to Blue-tie at once, recognizing the colour of the Blue-water school, and avoiding the absolute control and repression typified by black. But that would have spoilt the story, and prevented the disclosure of the qualities of the two men. When Blue-tie so utterly gave himself away to the girl, it was quite enough for the old negro. A Forsyte never does that. A Forsyte is thoroughly businesslike; honest too, but this idealism can twist the letter from the spirit to his own advantage—a triumph of the conscious.

The Virginian's idea of a contract is something different. He thinks not so much of the letter of

the bond as what it means to the other party.
He promised himself to this woman. It is a
personal, not a documentary relationship. He
is other-conscious.

He also has a pride of place. Our old aristocrats called themselves *ethelings*, and *ethel* in the
Arabic tongue, which is nearer our argument than
many imagine, means "rooted." The long-
heads are autochthonous, and realise it. It is
another aspect of Mediterranean character well
brought out in "The Skin Game"—which
brings us to Mr. Galsworthy and important
issues.

Mr. George Calderon, in his admirable preface
to *Two Plays of Tchekof*, furnishes a key to the
comprehension of Russian literature, whose
arbitrary realism so puzzles the English reader.
You think of Wordsworth's definition, "the
spontaneous overflow of powerful feeling";
you find it in Dostoievsky; but you miss the
recollection in tranquillity. There seems to be
no control at all. Mr. Calderon explains all this
very beautifully and makes a reference to Mr.
Galsworthy and his clear-cut distinctions—" the
wicked rich " and the suffering, perhaps deserving
poor. In English literature we have our clear-
cut villains and heroes. Why? They hardly

occur in real life. Yet we have an idea that men can help being bad or good; we are great believers in Free Will. That is it—the Asiatic Will again. We praise a man or condemn him; we don't look into his background, his parentage, his environment. We realize only the conscious, and neglect or condemn the unconscious. A similar outlook tends to mar Mr. Lay's useful book, *Man's Unconscious Conflict*. The conscious, being the moral and intellectual, is glorified; the unconscious is treated as a disease and a disgrace. Possibly Freud's pathological work, through being misunderstood, has done not a little to set people on the wrong track.

This Free Will attitude is not only manifest in our judgments, but also in the structure of literature. The Russian plot wanders on as if it could not help it. That is no excuse to an Englishman. A man *must* help it, whether in his life or his writing. Conscious control is demanded; a story must not maunder on; the author has got to keep it in check, plan it out, see that it arrives at a proper conclusion. This attitude towards a plot reflects the attitude towards life, and we have again the difference between Protestant and Catholic. The one feels that he can control life; the other that life is too much for him. It is the Asiatic contrasted with the Mediterranean point of view—the one with God in the cupboard, the other with God unapproachable ; the one above God, the other below Him.

This Catholic spirit pervades Russian literature, just as it pervaded Greek. *Anagke* was too much for the Greeks. It was their real complex,—the Oedipus complex being but a minor pathological one. They were up against Fate, Necessity, Life, forces greater than themselves. They worked off their feelings in their plays.

This attitude makes them kinder than we should have been. Helen brought untold woe to the world, but she is never condemned out and out. We are made to feel that she could'nt help it, poor woman ; her beauty was not her fault. We are not allowed to admire the bravery of heroes, nor the villainy of ruffiians ; for we see the gods pulling the strings all the time. That is what makes Greek legend so strange to us, perhaps so unreal. We want our heroes to be good and our villains to be bad on their own. We want an eye for an eye and a tooth for a tooth. Gradually we are beginning in our literature to realise that, if not the gods, there is

yet something behind these individual characters.
We are becoming more Catholic and merciful,
as the Asiatic yoke is lifted.

This is the key to Russian Literature. It is
realised that there is something behind, and so
the individual does not count for so much.
Tchekof expresses group emotions, his characters
act in a group. He tries to give you life itself.
No Englishman ventures to do this, because he
would seem to be missing his duty. He has to
show life under control—his own control. And
if he sees nothing behind life he can do this.
The plot is in his hands and he can serve it up
as he will.

I wish to close the chapter by a reference to
John Galsworthy, not as the portrayer of the
Wicked Rich, but of the eternal duality. He
perhaps more than any writer has developed that
threefold conflict of male and female, Asiatic and
Mediterranean, conscious and unconscious. And
for that reason, apart from its splendid literary
merits, *The Man of Property*—to single out one
in particular—is a book for all time. Possibly
Mr. Galsworthy himself realises this, for although
he never mentions these aspects, which seem to
be subconscious, he still continues to add to the
theme. He cannot drop the Forsytes.

It is a simple story of a beautiful, mystery woman, a fragile, uncertain, tender thing, something exquisitely beautiful and eternally feminine, wedded to a thorough-going Man of Property. This is nothing of the wicked rich about it. The writer feels the theme too great for that. Soames could not help it ; he behaved just as most Englishmen would have behaved, and our judges would have commended him. He exercised his marital rights.

Irene had been worried into this marriage, for she never loved Soames ; but she did her best for him until the right man came along—a man of her own race. It often happens that in a racially mixed marriage one of the parties reverts to its own racial type. There is first the natural tendency to variety, nature drawing opposites together for her own purposes ; but, that purpose accomplished, she lets them return to their own again. Irene reverted to Bosinney, the Buccaneer, the poor devil of an architect, who slept in his office. But what a house he built, and how he made Soames' money fly !

We are rather sorry for Soames, for he really loved his wife. He forgot that he promised her freedom if she should require it. All's fair in love and war, and a man who is really in love

will forget anything ; he will get the woman he
wants if he swings for it. After he had broken
into his wife's room, when she really belonged to
another man, he was very sorry. We are really
lifted into Catholic atmosphere. He was not at
fault ; it was his sense of property, his Asiaticism
that made him do it. He could not have acted
differently, nor could Irene, nor could Bosinney ;
they are just symbols of the duality of nature.
Old Jolyon would not have broken in like that,
nor would young Jolyon ; but then both had a
streak of the Hamite. Old Jo hated these men
of property, and loved women and little children ;
his son painted pictures and ran away with a
governess.

The tragedy is simple, not much in itself ;
it is almost an everyday affair. But the setting
is superb, utterly racial. " When a Forsyte died
—but no Forsyte had as yet died ; they did not
die ; death being contrary to their principles."

Swithin, " his shaven, square old face."

" Through the varying features an expression
of those fine forces could be marked, a certain
steadfastness of chin, underlying surface distinctions, marking a racial stamp."

" 'Phil never knows what he's got on ! ' No
one had credited an answer so outrageous.

A man not to know what he had on ?   No, no ! "

" Opportunists and egotists one and all."

" The position of their houses was of vital importance to the Forsytes, nor was this remarkable, since the whole spirit of their success was embodied therein."

" They collected pictures too, and were supporters of such charitable institutions as might be beneficial to their sick domestics.   From their father, the stone-mason, they inherited a real talent for bricks and mortar.   Originally, perhaps, members of some primitive sect, they were now in the natural course of things members of the Church of England."

" In that great London, which they had conquered and become merged in, what time had they to be sentimental ?"

" It was pleasant to think that in the after life he could get more for things than he had given."

" He had worked at that business !   Men did work in those days !   These young pups hardly knew the meaning of the word.   He had gone into every detail, known everything that went on, sometimes sat up all night over it."

" Old Jolyon was too much of a Forsyte to praise anything freely ; especially anything for which he had a genuine admiration."

" With his white head and dome-like forehead, the representative of moderation, and order, and love of property."

" Devising how to round off his property and make eternal the only part of him that was to remain alive."

Then Soames and his wife.

" The profound, subdued aversion which he felt in his wife was a mystery to him, and a source of the most terrible irritation. That she had made a mistake and did not love him, had tried to love him and could not love him, was obviously no reason."

" That she was one of those women—not too common in the Anglo-Saxon race—born to be loved and to love, who when not loving are not living, had certainly never even occurred to him."

" Soames had never called Irene an angel. He could not so have violated his best instincts, letting other people into the secret of her value, and giving himself away."

" Skin-like immaculateness had grown over Soames, as over many Londoners ; impossible to conceive of him with a hair out of place, a tie deviating one-eighth of an inch from the perpendicular, and collar unglossed ! He would not have gone without a bath for worlds—it was the fashion to take baths ; and how bitter was his scorn of people who omitted them !

But Irene could be imagined, like some nymph, bathing in wayside streams, for the joy of the freshness, and of seeing her own fair body."

The conflict does not end with *The Man of Property*. As the saga of the Forsytes continues we see that they represent England of the domination, so dear to Soames, which alas ! he sees passing away before his eyes to give place to the motor-car and the flapper. His thoughts on Mafeking night are interesting ! " They were hysterical—it wasn't English ! Restraint, reserve ! Those qualities to him more dear than life, those indispensable attributes of property, and culture, where were they ? It wasn't English !....It was as if he suddenly caught someone cutting the covenant ' for quiet possession ' out of his legal documents ; or of a monster lurking and stalking out in the future, casting its shadow before. Their want of solidity, their want of reverence ! It was like discovering that nine-tenths of the people of England were foreigners."

Precisely. They were awakening to the fact that they were Mediterraneans.

CHAPTER VI

THE SIGNIFICANCE OF THE SHORT-HEADS

I

I have worked on the assumption that the extreme type of Asiatic is the Mongol, an assumption not entirely recognized, and for which I will later state my grounds. We know his features, high cheek bones, oblique eyes, squat nose, lank black hair, and yellowish tint. Part of the Hittites of old were of this type, wearing pigtails and looking like Chinamen. The same types are seen in Brittany to-day, especially in Pont l'Abbé. There are little pools of Mongols left lying about Europe, and they are even to be met with in our own country. Topinard held the Breton eyes to be Asiatic ; de la Bourdonnais and Renan thought the Bretons mongoloid. In his *Races of Europe* Ripley tells us how the *homo alpinus* spread over Europe, and has since gradually receded to the mountains. Did the ebbing tide leave little pools behind ? Personally I think so. The Bigoudens of Brittany are regarded askance by their neighbours ; they have a style of art of their own, bizarre and angular, like the gipsy or Turkish. Their psychology and habits remind us of the Hittites.

Professor Keith, approaching the subject from his intimate knowledge of anatomy, takes a different view. Mongolism is a disease, common enough to-day. A defective thyroid will produce a mongol ; stunting growth, giving a yellow tinge to the skin, flattening the nose between the eyes, bulging the forehead, telescoping the face, causing the brain to act in a peculiar and aberrant manner. The first traditional Mongol was Japhet and Mr. Hrroabin's Japhet of the *Daily News* has most of the racial characteristics, physical and mental.

Professor Keith's address to the British Association in 1919 is full of interest. Our evolutionists are more and more inclined to adopt the view that nature progresses experimentally, and in this connexion we must necessarily be impressed by the work of the glands in the human body, for it is through the medium of these glands that Nature seems to experiment. According to Professor Keith the pituitary causes giantism and acromegaly, giving the European his height, his brow ridges and well-defined nose and chin. The suprarenal glands affect man's colour. Vagaries of the thyroid are responsible for mongolism, the features of which have been described. The face becomes crushed up and we get what is scientifically known as the bull-dog breed, a form of cretinism.

We know more than we realise. Whatever our bodily characteristics may be at the present day, we in this country are dominated by the Asiatic culture—I mean Puritanism, Public School, sport, and things of that kind. Accordingly we are well aware, quite apart from anything any scientist may tell us, that we are of the bull-dog breed. On our patriotic posters we depict an eminent sailor side by side with a bull-dog and could forgive the uninitiated for asking which is which. Our men of action, our popular heroes, are of the bull-dog breed, both mentally and facially. This is one of the things we know apparently by intuition—part of our general fund of unconscious knowledge.

Professor Keith holds that European mongols are local products and asserts that there is no evidence of a Turanian or Mongol invasion of

G

Europe in ancient times. This assertion is, however, contrary to archæological knowledge. The address following Sir Arthur Keith's is by Mr. Harold Peake, and deals with various Mongolian invasions of Europe commencing with the retreat of the ice-sheet. It is to these invasions that we owe the Lapps and the Finns.

The matter in this case is clinched by language, for there is a duality in language as in race. The language of the Mediterranean Race has become Indoeuropean, and that of the Mongols is Altaic or Ugro-Finnic. Such a language is talked by Finns, Lapps, Turks and Asiatic Mongols generally. Its home is acknowledged to be Asiatic. People could not sprout up pathologically in various parts of the world, all developing an Altaic language.

Owing to the erroneous view that Sanskrit represented a primitive type, and to the misunderstandings about skulls, the Indoeuropean languages are still supposed to have originated in Asia. Skeat says that philology depends on history ; but, if our history changes, so must our philology. The Indoeuropean languages are not Asiatic but African. If you examine the word *ear* in Skeat, you will find that he takes it back to a hypothetical type AUZON and leaves it there. He does not seem to have recognized that *auzon* is the Arabic for *ear*. This is not an isolated instance. Generally speaking, Skeat's hypothetical types are Arabic words, as I hope some day to demonstrate fully. Arabic is derived from the Hamitic of North Africa, a half-way house being Ancient Egyptian.

As the Mongols talked Mongolian, it is more than probable that they come from the home of Mongolians, Asia ; and this conclusion agrees with Sergi's. His short-headed man is marked by oblique eye-sockets, and other Mongolian features.

This conclusion does not exclude the fact that mongols may arise locally in a pathological manner. It merely shows that there is a great mongolism and a small mongolism, and we are considering the great—the Asiatic race which invaded Europe, one of whose features was mongolism.

Whatever Professor Keith's views may be on the origin of mongoloid peoples, there appears to be little doubt that they are pathological, as indeed every variation from the normal is held to be. Man began as a long-headed creature and ends as one. I have referred to the results of Beddoe's observations, and to the absorbent powers of the long-heads; and, apart from obstretrical considerations, it is the function of woman to draw the race back to its origin. Men are centrifugal, but she is centripetal. The short head was an accident and her function is to wipe out accidents; she tends therefore to make the race once more long-headed.

All races are in a way pathological and experimental, the products of the glands—the negro, the Malay, the European and the Mongol. But when the shape of a head is changed from long to short, a definitely new type is produced. We know that a mountain habitat is apt to produce cretinism, and we can only surmise that a body of mankind, wandering from their southern cradle, became isolated by the Himalayas and Hindu Kush. They certainly acquired a very distinct type of mentality, something quite different from what had prevailed before their development. The earlier long-headed people were children of nature, emotional, keen-sighted, æsthetic, uncontrolled. The Greek was noted for his clear sight, and short-headed critics like H. S. Chamberlain say that his philosophy suffered thereby. To the thorough-going philosopher, philosophy is a thing of the pure intellect and is marred by the assistance of the senses. For that reason it never progresses, and is often contrary to commonsense.

The shortening of the head from back to front seems to have been compensated by an access to its height, and a development of the hemispheres of the brain. These are the home of the control-centres, and one of the characteristics of the new race was control. Moreover in the general contortion the eye-sockets were shifted, and we get the mongolian eye.

Good sight keeps one in touch with nature ; it has something in common with the animal. Poor sight and developed brain lead to mathematics, logic, philosophy, metaphysics ; the nemesis of the over-developed brain is swelledhead, not uncommon among short-headed peoples.

Just as a blind man is cut off, so these new peoples were cut off, both from nature and their fellow men. In *The Genius of the Gael* Dr. Sophie Bryant says : " An Irish crowd mobilizes with a swiftness and Irish politicians can co-operate unexpectedly with a rapidity embarassing to Governments." That is to say they are bound together in some subterranean manner ; they act in unison like a pack of animals. We know that news is spread in a similar manner among savage tribes. That is to say, before the development of the conscious, man is not so much an individual as part of a community; he is essentially part of nature itself. The unconscious spreads out indefinitely both in space and time, binding together the past, the future and the universe.

Short-headed man, in developing the intelligence, developed the conscious. He developed will, free-will and egotism. He cut down through the links which bound him to the general unconscious, and became, for good or ill, an individual. He set up his own gods and his own values. He weighed everything in his intelligence and acted as seemed well to him; he became independent. He knows what he wants, and generally gets it; whether what he gets is of any value to him is another question.

3

Although short-headed man in some degree cut himself adrift from the unconscious, he did not necessarily become an isolated unit. As he developed reason, he expanded the ideal content of his environment, and learnt to live accordingly. Actuated by no unselfish motives, he realized the penalties of immoral conduct without necessarily incurring them. Through him has developed our business system based on honesty and trust, not necessarily for the love of these virtues, but because honesty is the best policy.

We thus obtain the idea of morality, which in effect is often a mere convention, a subservience to Mrs. Grundy. That it is more convention than real morality is seen often enough to-day and the conflict is a favourite one with writers of fiction. Morally the basis of sexual union is love, but conventionally it is marriage. In Mr. Chapin's beautiful play, *The Marriage of Columbine*, we see an exaggerated instance of marriage being morally wrong, and the lack of it morally right.

This conventional code is really herd morality, the rules of the game for hunting in a pack. Owing to its origin it is often ruthless and cruel ; it always lags behind the ethical life of the individual ; but it is a necessary foundation for social life. We see from Ibsen's *Enemy of the People* that perfect individual morality is regarded as a social sin.

Nevertheless as social life appears to be a necessary step in man's development, herd morality seems to be so much to the good. Possibly in the final state the rules of the game may be thrown aside, save for one or two conventions such as keeping to the proper side of the road, and the players can be trusted to play the game without external rules.

Most races have some sort of herd complex and herd morality, but short-headed man, owing to his qualities of idealism, seems to have developed them to the highest degree. Notable are the Romans and their law, and very different are the Greeks. H. S. Chamberlain says the Roman tree ran all to wood while Greece was a bower of leaves.

When you idealize, you classify ; you abstract the principles of things ; you unify. And that is what the Romans did. They made a uniform code, differing in this respect from our own law, that it provided for all cases beforehand. It was *a priori*, ours is manufactured *ad hoc*. That is the difference between the short-headed and the long-headed system. Idealism has the wherewithal to plan beforehand, to build up a scheme. Materialism takes facts as it finds them.

Idealism, classification, led to unity. The Roman Empire was one and homogeneous, and it was here that Greece failed. Her states were always warring against one another, till the Macedonian conquered and made them one.

Greece was a leafy bower—individual beauty, individual poetry, individual philosophy.

In Rome we are told that anyone who tried to be better than his comrades was accounted a bad citizen. For this reason it has been poetically argued that Julius Cæsar fell. One great feature has been ascribed to Mongols and Romans alike, anonymity, sacrifice of the individual to the herd. It requires a great deal of control and repression to effect this. No Mediterranean can do it : Athens coruscates with names.

This anonymity is achieved through idealism. The reward is remote, impersonal, in the future, in the hands of God, not tangible but ideal. Some in a still higher idealism ask no compensation. Like the Stoics, they are good because a man owes it to himself to be good. Here we arrive at something transcendental, beyond the scope of race. But whatever the motives for the act, the direction of the act is often guided by herd morality. Thus great Romans sacrificed themselves for Rome. The truly wise would weigh whether it was right to sacrifice oneself even for one's country.

It is a character of the short-heads that they will sacrifice themselves blindly for their fatherland. It was so in Rome, in Japan, in Germany,

and among the Mongols ; these are cannon-
fodder peoples.

The long-heads fight best when their blood
is up. Under the influence of a great emotion
they exhibit the *élan* so characteristic of the
French. Losing all reason, they become for the
moment natural men actuated by a sole impulse.
With the English it is different. They seldom
lose their control or their reason ; they regard
war in a detached manner, much more so than a
game of football. Their letters home are fired by
no burning, single-minded patriotism. They are
external and joke about the most solemn and
serious things. They regard it all as a game.
Some think it a foolish game, but generally
speaking, they abide by the rules.

4

Psychologists tell us that the idealizing mind
is the classifying mind, and the classifying the
unifying. To classify is to realize oneness
running through variety. And so these short-
heads conceived the idea of unity, differing in
this way from the emotional and sensuous long-
heads. The sensuous person sees only variety,
for he is a mirror in which external objects are
reflected. The short-head was unsensuous ; he

was not a mirror, for his eyesight was defective. He made up for this by creating a world in his brain, an ideal world. If externals did not fit into it, he made them.

If a person creates a world it is necessarily a world of unity, and external objects were made to fit into that unity. Therefore instead of the polytheism of the Greeks we get the monotheism of the Protestants. The Catholics are not monotheists by any means, as Mark Twain amusingly observes.

But there was another force among the short-heads making for unity ; or perhaps it was part of the same force. The idealist is egotistical, and the short-heads were extremely so. Their point of view that they created creation shews it. Naturally creation included God, and in a way they created Him. At least they recognise no other than their own God, who is obviously themselves. The God of the Germans is the stern *Hausvater*, and the God of John Knox is a dominant male.

The God of the Old Testament is very much this kind of God, for he is really the basis. The Hebrews were originally an Arabic people, but they picked up most of their theology and folk-lore among their short-headed neighbours,

Armenians and Babylonians. There were numerous local gods in Palestine and Syria, against whom the prophets were constantly inveighing, and finally Jehovah prevailed. He was a patriarch like Abraham himself, the God of Abraham, Isaac and Jacob, dominating, arbitrary, even fickle, as they were. He was not above human weaknesses, and he showed a certain despotic capriciousness in the matter of the sacrifice of Isaac. Nor was he above a bargain, and in fact the whole basis of Old Testament religion was a bargain or covenant.

When our fathers used to take us to church or, even better, to chapel, they paraded the wife and family for the inspection of their God. Presbyterians and Dissenters loved long and wordy sermons, and the atmosphere of purity and righteousness ; it was the atmosphere of the Englishman's home. Women and children were there on sufferance, and were to learn to keep in their places.

Catholics go to church in a very different spirit, and men attend far less than women. The Catholic's attitude is one of submission. Realising himself as an inseparable part of the eternal he just goes to acknowledge his oneness and his smallness. *In la sua voluntade è nostra pace.*

The short-headed type of mind gives us not only unity, but absoluteness. For Asiatics were a male race, and came to Europe as dominating males, holding women and children in subjection. And as their lack of vision forced them into metaphysics, so their dominating nature drove them to find the Absolute. This is the basis of Hegelian philosophy, the greatest exposition of which is *Appearance and Reality*. But, however logically convincing, if we can understand it, this work may be, we must necessarily look with suspicion on anything touching the Absolute, since it is the product of the pathological Asiatic mind, a mind which, as Bertrand Russell says, did not realize relations, which did not recognise anything external to itself. To the author of this work the world as we see it is merely appearance ; with this we may contrast the view of the neo-Hamite philosopher, Bergson, that things are what they appear to be. The first is contrary to common-sense ; the latter in accordance with it. To the Hegelian truth lies only in the fiction of his own idealism, the Absolute.

The Mediterraneans had that concreteness of the imagination which distinguished Keats. They were concrete in their ideas, sensuous, sense-impressionist, materialist. It was the

short-heads who invented abstraction. Starting
from the idea the brachycephals built up a world
which had its origin in the ego. Their ego was
supreme.

The response of the long-head to his environment is direct and natural, but with the short-
head the environment is modified by the ideal
content. The response may be to the ideal content alone. As this is largely compounded of the
ego, both will and hope are emphasized. Jacque
Vontade says the English are unmatched hopers,
which is to say that we have strong self-regarding
wishes. The will, whatever be its place in the
new psychology, has always been a characteristic
of the short-heads.

I suppose in the light of Freud and Holt we
ought to revise our view of the will. Perhaps
we may regard it as a permanent response to the
ideal environment, which is dominated by the
ego. The legal will, the will *par excellence*,
whereby the state acknowledges the projection
of a man's personality beyond death, was given
us by the Romans—an extraordinary concession
to the personal ego.

Perhaps one of the most outstanding features
of the short cranium is its powerof co-ordination ;
it is essentially the co-ordinating head, giving

self-control which leads to the power of controlling others. There is probably a simple physiological explanation of this phenomenon. The brain is like a telephone exchange in which the nerve endings are temporarily juxtaposed. Where any nerves may have to be placed in touch with any other, obviously the most convenient shape for the exchange is a circle rather than an ellipse. But whatever be the explanation, the short-head is the better co-ordinated. This is brought out most particularly in games. Both long and short-headed peoples excel in games, but, as we have seen, in games of a different kind.

CHAPTER VII

DUALITY IN PSYCHOLOGY

I

Conscious and unconscious to-day are terms which have gained both in precision and significance largely owing to the work of the Freudians, and, in referring to the two races as being of the conscious and unconscious type, it must be understood that I am speaking broadly. Both peoples are equipped in the normal way with a mind which is both conscious and unconscious, and in calling one people conscious and another unconscious it is merely intended to signify that with one the conscious qualities predominate and with the other the unconscious. As we probe more deeply into the psychological aspects of the subject it will be necessary to consider more closely the nature of the conscious and unconscious, and to indicate how and why short-headed man is of the conscious type.

We are at present treating the subject inductively, reasoning from facts rather than principles, and I want to make a fairly complete picture of these facts before entering into the why and the wherefore. Our survey of races, ancient and modern, has indicated the existence of two very distinct types ; psychologists, dealing with all heads and not any particular kind of head, have also discovered that people ordinarily fall into two types. It will be observed after perusal that these are no other than our long and short-headed types.

2

Dr. Geley (*From the Unconscious to the Conscious*), presents the types in the following manner. In the first " the centralisation is strong and the homogeneity obvious. The central monad—the self—directs the mental dynamo-psychism, and has complete control over all its elements. Through the mental dynamo-psychism it directs the vital dynamism and the body.... The individual, so constituted, is in stable equilibrium. His psychic health is perfect. But at the same time he finds himself severely limited by organic conditions. The solidarity of his superior psychism with his central psychism being absolute all the activities of the former are limited by the extent of the latter and restrained within its conditions.

" Such an individual cannot be conscious of his latent powers, nor of anything which concerns his higher psychism. In him the products of higher inspiration and of his brains are closely unified and make a harmonious whole. His psychology is *normal*—typical—marked by the equilibrium of his faculties and their regular output, but also by their narrow limitations.

" . . . . There are among them many mediocrities but also some very intelligent men. Their intellectual output is regular and contains no surprises. . . . they know nothing of intuition ; they are never original. If they understand art they are never artists in the higher sense of the word ; still less are they inventors or creative. They have no genius, and none of the higher kind of inspiration.

" Well balanced minds play a useful part in science and social life by their poise and the correctness of their reasoning on ordinary matters ; they are also detrimental by their hatred of innovation and their immovable attitude."

In the unstable individual on the other hand,

" contrariwise to what we have noted in the well-balanced men, we find a want of homogeneity and dependence between the different constituent principles. The centralising direction is imperfect ; there is no harmonious fusion between the self and the mentality, between the mentality and the vital dynamism, and between this last and the organism.

" This state of unstable equilibrium allows of momentary and partial decentralisations, which are indeed sources of disorder but are also conditions in which the lessened limitations imposed by the body allow of the possibility of bringing to light everything which in the normal psyhic being is cryptoid and occult, whether of the nature of faculty or of knowledge. But this manifestation is never regular ; the intellectual output is occasional and spasmodic ; it requires a collaboration of the conscious and the subconscious ; and the modalities and difficulties of this collaboration are well known.

" There are among them mediocrities, in whom, however, a tinge of originality corrects psychological monotony.

" There are inferior neuropaths who drag out a morbid existence of semi-insanity and semi-imbecility, showing the mental and physical defects which are now called degeneracy.

" There are also superior neuropaths whose talents or genius are inseparable from similar defects. These defects cause great suffering ; the superior neuropath finds it hard to govern his grouping, or direct his body and even his mentality. Often his mentality escapes more or less from his control and he then skirts the edge of total disequilibrium or insanity.... He feels dimly the limitations imposed on him by his nerves and brain.....

" How much suffering is involved in these limitations, in the intuitive perceptions of genuine intuitive faculty, which nevertheless are not at his free disposal ; in the desire to reduce large abstract perceptions to concrete analytical work ; in the effort to express in words that which he conceives so well without words ; in the necessity which obliges him to submit the work of his highest and conscious self to the lower organic mechanism.

"Another type of neuropath not less curious than the man of genius is the medium.... The medium is not master in his own house....he is extremely impressionable ; he is very suggestible ; he is very unstable in his temper and ideas."

Mr. Tansley's *New Psychology* offers us a similar pair of psychological types.

" The other pair of contrasted types of mentality is that described by Trotter in his very valuable work on the psychology of the herd instinct, as the *stable-minded* and the *unstable-minded* types. The stable-minded or resistive type is to be regarded as the normal type among primitive peoples. The possessor of this kind of mind is full of energy and activity and of strong will relatively resistent to the effects of experience. His opinions on most topics are relatively fixed, and he is generally contented and of a placid disposition. He has a number of well-marked complexes with well-defined channels allowing of the strong and smooth outflow of psychic energy. The possessor of a stable mind, therefore, fits well into its place in the social organism. In the complex modern societies he still exists in large numbers, and notably among the governing classes. The rigid organization of his mind makes him relatively insensitive to experience of a type that cannot easily be dealt with and assimilated to his fixed and stable complexes. He is inadaptable and ill-fitted to cope with the rapid and far-reaching changes which are taking place in the structure and spirit of the modern world. The regular soldier of the " old school " is perhaps the most typical and extreme example of stable-mindedness, but the same type is met with among many classes of society which pursue old and well-established modes of life, for instance among clergymen, country squires, and government officials.

" The unstable-minded type, on the other hand, has the opposite characters. Its great positive quality is extreme sensitiveness to varied experience, and this facility of reaction naturally carries with it the characteristic instability. Weak will and want of persistence are marks of this type. The opinions of the unstable-minded man are often heterodox, and he is rarely consistently happy or contented. He has constantly shifting mental complexes, and therefore ill-defined conative channels. The extremely unstable-minded person is often of the type known as " decadent," and is then unsparingly condemned by the stable-minded. He would find short shrift in a primitive society, but the security, variety of conditions, and formal tolerance existing in modern civilized societies enables him to survive and it seems probable that he is actually fast multiplying in numbers.

The great merit of the unstable mind is flexibility and adaptability to new conditions, and for this reason it has a general intellectual superiority to the stable type. The unstable-minded man is often charged with immorality, owing to his frequent refusal to be bound by the opinions and lines of action laid down by society, but his ethical sense may, in fact, be highly developed, though his morality is likely to be experimental. The real weakness of the unstable mind is its changeableness, which commonly renders its possessor unsafe to depend upon and rarely capable of the prolonged effort necessary to considered achievement."

These types are not merely psychological abstractions. We meet them in everyday life, and I doubt whether we really meet anything else. We all know our Forsyte, our Man of Property, who goes through life laying brick upon brick, coin upon coin, methodical, thrifty, trustworthy, a man of character. He generally takes a bath, is clean of person, has his hair cut regularly, dresses quietly but well. Square of face, powerful in the jaw, with good teeth, he does not look a man to be trifled with. If he has a physical weakness it is generally in the eyes; that is the ransom he has to pay. He eats well, but sees badly ; visual sense has suffered at the expense of brain development. He is no intuitionist, and does not see a joke ; you must explain it to him. He reconstructs it word by word, and often the poor joke, the love-child of intuition, is lost in the mass of masonry. And so the extreme type of our John Bull is the Lowland Scot. It is the same with dancing, to which he never takes naturally ; he must work it all out intellectually and mathematically, and therefore, missing the intuition and sympathy of the art, he will never dance.

Very methodical, even meticulous, he despises rough and ready methods. He has no marks for artist-chaps, musicians, mountebanks. His scope may not be very wide, but he thoroughly covers it. Though he may not achieve overwhelming success, his methods do not allow him to fail ; he is the typical merchant or shopkeeper.

He is seldom ill, for he can control things of that sort. He is no victim of the emotions. Though he misses the raptures of joy, he also avoids the depths of despair. On the whole he is the happiest man on earth, for everything is subject to his control ; and if it is not, he imagines it is, and is happy. In this way he is an idealist. He can call black white or do a questionable action without turning a hair. If it is not right, he makes it right.

Protestantism appeals to him ; if he is not a Dissenter, he finds the Low Church near enough to dissent for his purpose. He likes a good sermon appealing to the intellect or inculcating the morality of the house-father. He will have no truck with vestments, incense, candles, miracles, ornaments, or other paraphernalia of the Scarlet Woman. His God is the prototype of himself, master in his own household, keeping women and children in their proper places.

In politics he inclines to Liberalism, for he is a descendant of the old Whigs, and, before them, of the Roundheads. This does not mean that he is a progressive. Liberalism appeals to him because of its intellectualism and common-sense.

For education he has a great respect, however little of it he possesses himself. But his son shall do better. He likes good sound reading, with plenty of words ; a leader in *The Times* or *The Observer* ; a long article is like a big building or a large picture ; you get plenty for your money.

An efficient, sound, moral citizen.

Your other man is a bit of a vagabond, dining indiscriminately at the Carlton or behind a hedge-row. He wears his hair long, and his collar short—a regular Bosinney. He has very good eyes, which flash and sparkle. He makes jokes and enjoys them. Perhaps he hardly makes them—they come. They represent the unconscious welling up in him. Sometimes he is a genius, sometimes a hopeless failure, but he is always lovable. He is fond of children and loves women—often not wisely but too well. A dancer, a poet, a Bohemian, an artist, we are in doubt sometimes whether we can trust him, or take him seriously. But beneath his nonsense there are flashes of truth ; we suspect him of pulling our leg. He reaches to the heights and the depths both of knowledge and emotion, he is in the clouds or in hell. For a night of rapture he will starve for weeks, or ruin himself eternally ; Cleopatra is worth the Nile. An unstable, emotional fellow, catabolic. Yet we feel we must recognise his value in sounding the heights and the depths for us—a *ballon d'essai.*

Perhaps he likes reading, but it is out-of-the-way stuff—Swinburne, astrology, heraldry, Greek vases. Or perhaps he does not read, knowing already. He does not have to build up his knowledge—a phrase, an image, a flash, will convey all he wants to know, for he has such good eyes. That is how he takes things in, like the Greeks; he is an intuitionist.

He is often distrusted, for he gets hold of a truth and can't prove it. He merely knows it; but John Bull demands proof, something in black and white.

Generous and unselfish, he often ends in beggary. His life is outside himself—in others or in nature. He is other-conscious.

In religion either a Catholic or an agnostic. Catholicism appeals to him by its sensuousness, or because of his own weakness and instability. But if he is strong enough, his sense of humour will not tolerate religion. He is naturally a rebel and will not go to Church even if it is only because other people go.

His politics shew the same extremes. Emotionalism tends to bind him to the past; he is part of the eternal; and so he may be a conservative; but not necessarily. As in the Irishman, his extreme type, this sense of continuity may carry him into the future, or beyond the realms of fact and possibility. He may be a revolutionist, demagogue, labour leader, Sinn Feiner, Bolshevist. Since he is free of the ego, his suggestibility and emotionalism may carry him far.

He is not hard-headed or brainy and, indeed,

his intellect may be defective. But he is often brilliant, always original and defiant of authority.

An untrustworthy fellow, but it would not be much of a world without him.

It will be observed that Geley's types are much the same as Tansley's or Trotter's and also the same as my own. The last are definitely racial; Geley's are in a special sense conscious and unconscious. Whether your division is racial or psychological the result is the same, and that is our justification for regarding Asiatics and Mediterraneans as conscious and unconscious.

Geley, finding our theories of evolution inadequate, postulates a dynamo-psychism behind it, planning, directing. This is a single force, the ultimate life-force, the unconscious. Personality is but its representation in the conscious world; individuals are like commercial travellers representing their firm in a town. We are individual representatives, but we belong to and represent one firm; our nature is in that way dual. Such a conception fits very well into our scheme of the races. One traveller may be a mere representative, having no mind, no interest, beyond that of his firm. Life may thus be difficult for him, for he has to adapt himself to his surroundings, to fit in with his city, his

customers. He has his own life to lead, and this
may conflict with absolute devotion to his firm.
On the other hand he has a certain strength in
the mutual loyalty between himself and his firm.
He has all their wealth and power behind him.
The chief danger is that in the representative
the man may be lost. Business, like life,
develops, and even the strongest firm may not
last for ever. Such a person is the Mediterranean.

Some travellers are not so loyal. Equipped
by their firm they may start businesses on their
own, displaying their independence but renounc-
ing their allegiance. They prefer to carry on
their work as individuals. They may meet with
success or failure. Success brings freedom and
independence, but it can never be a very great
success, and it may be entirely illusory, for an
individual's resources are trifling compared with
those of a powerful firm. But such a person has
for good or ill chosen independence, and he must
abide by it. Such a type is the Asiatic.

Among his unconscious types, Geley includes
mediums, neuropaths, and others more or less
mentally defective or abnormal and, in order to
include these, perhaps we ought to alter our
imagery somewhat. Suppose we regard the
conscious as a cap. Beneath it are the unlimited

and extensive powers of the dynamo-psychism, the unconscious. In the stable type, the Asiatic, the cap fits well, entirely covering, controlling, possibly extinguishing, the unconscious. With the medium, the neuropath, or the Mediterranean, the cap fits badly; it is too small and does not cover the unconscious, or it is on one side and leaves part of the unconscious uncovered. Phenomena of mediumism, prophecy, second-sight, impulsive and inconsidered action, are instances of the unconscious emerging to the surface.

We may look at the question in still another way. Imagine a flat surface of molten material, rising into numerous bubbles, which may represent our individuals. These bubbles are part of the mass and yet they are bubbles. They have solidarity with the magma, which is the unconscious. On the other hand some of the bubbles may dry off and become separated from the surface. They now have individual freedom, they are entities; but their freedom has been gained at the expense of solidarity with the whole and of the strength which they drew as parts of it. This is another aspect of the Mediterranean and the Asiatic.

CHAPTER VIII

SEX DUALITY.

I

Having indicated the parallelism of racial and psychological duality, we will now proceed to consider the more obvious duality of sex, and we can readily accomplish this with Mr. Havelock Ellis' *Man and Woman* as a guide.

We find that woman's work is of a general and routine character; it is man who is the specialist. Women excel in activities of a routine character.

As for love-making, in the early epics it is woman who is the wooer the man being indifferent and less sensual.

The young ape is nearer to man than the old ape; mankind is descended from the young ape. In the same way woman is nearer the child, and the child is probably, from an evolutionary point of view, a higher type than the adult. Foetal evolution is in an upward direction ; development after birth is mere adaptation. Woman in her retention of child characteristics represents both the past and the future. She thus partakes of the eternal. Man specializes, varies, experiments ; the race can adopt his successes and avoid his failures.

" The man's form is erect and closely knit, the woman's is more uneven, with large hips and flowing protuberant curves of breast and abdomen and flanks. While the man's form seems to be instinctively seeking action, the woman's falls naturally into a state of comparative repose, and seems to find satisfaction in an attitude of overthrow."

" During the development of puberty girls of the European race are both taller and heavier than boys of the same age." " The evolution of puberty is more precocious in girls than in boys." And though more boys are born than girls, they are harder to rear ; one may suggest, because they are experimental. The preponderance of boys over girls at birth is most striking in Greece and the so-called Celtic fringes of Britain. The Registrar General supposed the reason, as regards Britain, to be racial, but Mr. Havelock Ellis cannot see any foundation for the view.

In the light of Freud the reason may indeed be racial. In creating a son, a woman is creating a lover ; and the Mediterranean women would miss no opportunity.

Some are of opinion to-day that woman is becoming more masculine. Physically this is not the case. The pelvis is the cradle of the child, and a broad pelvis indicates strong maternity. The pelvis in the ape and in primitive races is narrow ; with civilisation it becomes broad ; and man's pelvis tends to broaden towards the woman's. I might remark that the wide pelvis is a Mediterranean and not an Asiatic trait. The short-headed tradition is for women to be straight up and down like a boy. This is a tendency of Greek statuary, and it is emphasized by the *chiton*. But the eternal woman, the evolutionary woman, is the sinuous Mediterranean.

We find some anthropologists asserting that in Europe women are more dolichocephalic than men ; others that they are more brachycephalic ; and both may be right. Where dolichocephaly is original women will tend to be more dolichocephalic ; where brachycephaly, more brachycephalic. For woman is always drawing the race back to its origins.

In Europe we find that " men possess
absolutely larger brains than women." The
intellect, like man himself, is more or less of an
accident or an experiment. Man's characteristic is intelligence, woman's intuition.

The female sex is anabolic, acquiring rather
than expending ; males are catabolic and
wasteful.

We find that women are more sensitive to pain
than men. We should naturally expect in them
a greater sensuous than intellectual development. For some reason, however, man has a
keener sense of smell. This is possibly, because
our sense of smell has become artificial. A
woman may sense a smell without knowing it.
Man appears to excel in distinguishing smells,
which is a different thing.

Similarly in taste, hearing and sight, men
appear to have the advantage. The reasons are
probably the same, for men specialize in artificial
distinctions. On the other hand such entirely
emotional faculties as coloured hearing, coloured
associations, are far more developed in woman.

" Women reveal everywhere a somewhat less
capacity for motor energy than men and a less
degree of delight in its display." Like the sphinx
woman sits and smiles, while man displays his

fireworks.   The only exception is dancing, which
is of course woman's sex-advertisement.   As
regards direction of motion, woman's, whether in
buttoning garments or any other activity, tends
to be from right to left, man's from left to right.
That is, she is centripetal, while man is centrifugal.   Woman appears to be less skilful with
her hands.   This seems strange, at first, but it
must be remembered that manual dexterity is
specialized.   In normal activities, as well as in
most normal functions, woman is superior.   She
remains at the fountain-head.

We find that, when people are asked to write
down quickly a certain number of words, women
specialize on dress and foods—the ultimate
essentials of the *libido*.   " In general," says
Professor Jastrow, " the feminine traits revealed
by this study are an attention to the immediate
surroundings, to the finished product, to the
ornamental, the individual, and the concrete ;
while the masculine preference is for the more
remote, the constructive, the useful, the general,
and the abstract."

" The masculine method of thought is massive
and deliberate, while the feminine method is
quick to perceive and nimble to act.   The latter
method is apt to fall into error, but is agile in

retrieving an error and under many circumstances this agility is the prime requirement. Whenever a man and a woman are found under compromising circumstances it is nearly always the woman who, with ready wit, audaciously retrieves the situation..... It is unnecessary to insist on this quality, which in its finest forms is called tactfulness." Here again we are led to think of " Scotch " and " Irish " characters.

Buckle noticed that the wit of woman starts from ideas rather than from the patient collection of facts ; from this he came to the erroneous conclusion that men were inductive and woman deductive. Of course the reverse is the case. Havelock Ellis corrects the opinion by saying that " women start more readily, perhaps without any conscious intellectual process, from the immediate fact before them." That is, they react as a whole, and intuitively, like the Irish. Personally, I have a very good recollection of faces, but I can never describe a person's features. The face strikes me as a whole, and that is how woman re-acts.

Woman is of course no metaphysician, but, for some reason, she attains to distinction in mathematics. My experience is that woman is either no mathematician at all, or else she is a good one.

Mr. Havelock Ellis has some difficulty in accounting for the paradox of woman's superiority in this field. He explains it, and perhaps correctly, by suggesting that the fact is due to woman's docility and receptiveness. As Burdach said, " Women take truth as they find it, while men want to create truth."

Mathematics has this peculiarity, that it is all there. You have only got to follow, for it simply says " Come and find me." On the other hand, mathematical women are few, and their success in this abstract science may be due to exceptional maleness in their constitution.

Possibly, however, there is another solution, that mathematics is ultimately a machine, and, though women may not be skilful at making machines, they excel in using them.

In their philosophic tastes we find that " women are attracted to the most concrete of all abstract thinkers, to the most poetic, and the most intimately personal, and above all, to the most religious."

While women have done little in religious leadership, it has been remarked that they are probably more fitted for politics than men. Religious leadership is, I think, a contradiction of terms. The religious person is a follower, and that is what women are, resembling in this the Irish. As regards the priesthood of women, this has been impossible during Asiatic dominance, but in ancient days it was usual and is now being revived. Politics are merely economy, which is woman's province. My experience of women workers is that they are more practical than men. The male politician tends to be brilliant and catabolic. A man of genius is often a danger in politics.

"Women respond to stimuli, psychic and physical, more readily than men." They have greater affectability. That is, the response does not have to go through such a large conscious loop. They are more unconscious and animal. Woman's spontaneity is popularly referred to as tenderness of heart. Women blush more easily than men, their faces are more expressive and more mobile.

Primitive women have in their hands the rudiments of most of the arts. When we get past the rudiments we find the differentiated arts in the hands of men. This is partly because man is a specialist, partly because in primitive ages he had more time on his hands ; mainly because, while woman always has her domestic duties, man's natural tendencies are repressed, and the outlet for repression is art. There are his instincts sublimated.

" Music is at once the most emotional and the most severely abstract of arts. There is no art to which women have been more widely attracted, and there is certainly no art in which they have shewn themselves more helpless." This is a most important conclusion. Music is perhaps the most absolute form of art ; the most arbitrary, and the least rational. Yet its highest development is associatd with ages of rationalism and it is generally cultivated by the most intellectual races and individuals. We must conclude that it is the outlet *par excellence* for repression ; the great compensation to the over-developed conscious. Therefore women should not need it so much as men ; its abstraction runs contrary to their concrete nature ; and feminine nature lacks the necessary co-ordination for good execution. Probably women, like the Maltese, for instance, have a very musical nature ; but they fall short in execution.

On the other hand the abstractness of music may appeal to the male in the same way as the naturalness of mathematics appeals to the female.

" In poetry, women have done much more than

in either mysticism, or metaphysics....but it is difficult to find women poets who shew in any noteworthy degree the qualities of imagination, style, and architectural power which go to the making of great poetry." Probably the same arguments apply here as to music. Women suffers less repression and she has less co-ordination. " In fiction women are acknowledged to rank incomparably higher than in any other form of literary art." This is because fiction requires above all things concreteness of the imagination. " It is only when (as in the work of Flaubert) the novel almost becomes a poem, demanding great architectonic power, severe devotion to style, and complete self-restraint, that women have not come into competition with men." They excel in the unconscious and fail in the conscious.

" There is, however, one art in which women may be said not merely to rival but actually excel men; this is the art of acting." Their sympathy makes them throw themselves into a part, and to become it. They react concretely and as a whole.

" Ferrero has sought the explanation of the small part played by women in art, and their defective sense for purely æsthetic beauty, in their less keen sexual emotions." He evidently had great insight. It is the repression of sexualism which made man realize the world around him.

" Suicide in Europe is from three to four times more frequent in man than in woman." " Men hang themselves and women drown themselves." Havelock Ellis explains that women prefer passivity and hate to make a mess, but perhaps there is more in it than this. In that greatest of all crises mankind is perhaps not disinclined to fall back on eternal symbolism. Man belongs to the sky and the sun ; woman to the earth and the water. The root *ma* means both mother and water.

In insanity " causes acting on the brain are more common in men ; moral and sentimental causes are more common in women." " The criminal and anti-social impulse is less strong in women than in men."

There is a " greater general variability in the male sex." " Men have a greater tendency to abnormality than women." " Women represent the more stable and conservative element in evolution." " We have, therefore, to recognise that in men, as in males generally, there is an organic variational tendency to diverge from the average ; in women, as in females generally, an organic tendency, notwithstanding all their facility for minor oscillations, to stability and conservatism, involving a diminished individualism and variability."

"Men show a more marked variational tendency, and this fact is closely allied with the fact....that men exhibit more marked pathological characters ; for, as Vichow insists, every deviation from the normal type must have its foundation in a pathological accident."

"A large part of the joy that men and women take in each other is rooted in this sexual divergence in variability. The progressive and divergent energies of men call out and satisfy the twin instincts of women to accept and follow a leader, and to expend tenderness on a reckless and erring child, instincts often intermingled in delicious confusion. And in women men find beings who have not wandered so far as they have from the typical life of earth's creatures ; women are for men the human embodiments of the restful responsiveness of Nature. To every man, as Michelet has put it, the woman whom he loves is as the Earth was to her legendary son ; he has but to fall down and kiss her breast and he is strong again. Woman is more in harmony with Nature than man, as Burdach said, and she brings man into harmony with Nature. This organically primitive nature of women in form and function and instinct, is always restful to men tortured by their vagrant energies ; it was certainly with genuine satisfaction that the tender and sympathetic Diderot wrote of women that " they are real savages inside." It is because of this that the ascetics—those very erractic and abnormal examples of the variational tendency, have hated women with hatred so bitter and intense that no language could be found strong enough to express their horror. They knew that every natural impulse of a woman is the condemnation of asceticism. All true lovers of the artificial and perverse find women repulsive ; " Woman is natural," it is written among the sayings of Baudelaire, " that is to say abominable." But for most men and women this sexual difference has added to the charm of life ; it has also added to the everlasting difficulty of life."

Summing up, Mr. Havelock Ellis draws attention to the greater variability of the male, the greater precocity of women, the nearness of woman to the child-type ; she is conservative, yet represents the type to which man is approx-- mating. But her conservatism is cosmic and not

social.   It is like the Irishman's or the Catholic's.
It is a conservatism in harmony with nature and
the eternal, not with the retrograde and re-
actionary.

2

Male and female bodies are only shells for the
gametes, and in sex matters it is the gametes
which dominate.   Says Mr. Tansley in *The New
Psychology :* " The minute microscopic gametes
are the actual mating organisms ; the ' sexual'
features, both physical and mental, of the complicated bodies which, in the higher animals,
produce and perfect them till mating can be
accomplished—the sexual individuals of ordinary
language—are built up in relation to the primary
characters of these mating cells."

From the behaviour of the gametes we can
gain some insight into sex psychology. Mr.
Tansley continues :

" The sexual gametes are very unlike in every
respect. The male is small, very active, and
often very sensitive to chemical stimuli arising
from the female. The body of the male gamete
is, in fact, reduced to the smallest limits com-
patible with these qualities and with the carrying
of the substance necessary for a fertile mating...

The male gamete is short-lived, having no store of reserve food nor the power to nourish itself, and if it does not succeed in mating it soon dies."

" The female gamete, on the other hand, is relatively large, containing a quantity of stored food....and is quite passive so far as actual movement is concerned. An important part of its activity, however, is often the production of certain chemical substances which diffuse into the medium around it, and, reaching the male gametes, guide these to the female. Normally, only one male gamete mates with the female, and as soon as mating occurs the secretion of attractive substance is stopped."

It appears then that the function of the female is to sit still and attract ; having attained her object she ceases to attract.

The unconscious attitude of woman has been obscured by historical events. We are nearing the end of a period of male domination—an unnatural domination which is now disappearing as we revert to Mediterraneanism. Woman has been repressed, and many women, English women more than French, tend to be unnatural. After their harem-life they are necessarily uncertain of themselves. The natural woman betrays herself mainly in her unconscious. We

see "attractive lingerie" advertised in our
newspapers, and the most moral women do not
disdain it.   The most respectable women do not
refrain from displaying very attractive legs.   All
specialise in those highly electrical substances,
silk and hair.   The more Mediterranean women
emphasize their sexual allurements—the Cretans
of old and the Parisennes to-day.   Dress and
adornments are part of the armoury of the female
unconscious.   If a woman, passing a man in the
street, fancies that his glance has been too
insistent, she may shew her annoyance, but when
she has passed her hand almost invariably flies
to her hair.

Probably Pope had something of this in his
mind when he said that every woman is at heart
a rake.   However moral she may be consciously,
unconsciously she allures.   Nor do her unconscious delinquencies stop here.   The kiss is the
relic of a bite, and the sexual act of a devouring.
Insect life is full of tragedies of this kind ; the
female devours her mate as she enjoys him.
In *Susan Lenox*, the enraged Freddie Palmer
bursts out : " You've made a fool of me, as a
woman always does of a man.   If she loves him,
she destroys him.   If she doesn t love him, he
destroys himself."   In *Sex Antagonism* Mr.

Heape tells of a young girl of fourteen who, on being asked what she would like best in the world, replied that she would like to marry and have four children ; then she would like her husband to die and bring them up herself.

Woman is brim-full of the unconscious, and that makes her position in the conscious world somewhat difficult. For instance, when war breaks out, with its usual intense emotional concomitants, her unconscious is apt to run away with her. She likes to see her boy in khaki, and presents white feathers to those who are not. There is undoubtedly a deep-rooted unconscious antagonism between the sexes and I have often wondered whether this was an instance of it. I discussed the matter with one woman, and she told me that the reason was that woman wanted men to fight for her. But I am not altogether satisfied that this is conclusive.

Man's position towards woman is exceedingly delicate. She created her experiment—unconsciously she appears to control these things, for after a war there is always an increase in male births—and charged him with desire. Unconsciously she allures, consciously she repels. Having wound up his spring to breaking point she often turns him aside with a laugh, and the Sunday papers reap the benefit.

Her position is summed up in Goethe's *Harfenspieler* :

" Ihr führt ins Leben uns hinein,
    Ihr laszt den Armen schuldig werden,
    Dann überlaszt ihr ihn der Pein ;
    Denn alle Schuld rächt sich auf Erden.

As male domination recedes into the background this anomalous position of the male becomes more emphasized in literature. We have less of *Susan Lenox* and more of *The Black Diamond*.

3

Goethe probably had some inkling of the true state of the case when he spoke of *das ewige Weibliche*. The eternal feminine has a wider meaning than appears at first sight. It has a kind of implication that the feminine is the eternal. And that is in a sense true.

Life starts as unicellular and becomes multicellular. In the same way bisexualism is preceded by unisexualism. The union of single-celled organisms seems to be accidental in its origin. There was no particular difference between the uniting cells. " The mating of living cells," said Mr. Tansley, " to produce a new organism is not necessarily associated with

a difference of sex.   In many of the lowest forms
of life the pair of mating gametes are equivalent
in all respects."   We must suspect that the new
form of reproduction was accidental, and was
adopted by natural selection for its utility.   In
many ways cell-divisions are more satisfactory
than sexual mating, but the growing complica-
tion of the organism involved true sex.   An
elephant could not shed a leg to produce a new
elephant, and without sex-mating such a complex
thing as an elephant would have been impossible.

The subject is well treated in Geddes &
Thompson's *Sex*.   Sex mating appears to have
been necessary for developed life.   It provides
elasticity, a new start, and affords a protection
to the gametes.

The origin of the male is therefore humble.
Fortuitous, probably arising from hunger and
cannibalism ; an experiment, retained as useful ;
exceeding   all   dreams ;   a   *ballon d'essai*, a
pointer for the race.   When baulked of its
legitimate purpose, sublimating its desires in the
arts, useful and ornamental, in the realization of
nature, in contemplation, in idealism, in the
conscious.

The sex question is well illustrated by a study
of the bees.   The female workers control the

number and sex of the eggs. The queen has it
in her power to produce male or female eggs at
will. The drone egg is not fertilized ; the drone
is an incomplete female. The rigour of the
female unconscious is observed in this community. The drones enjoy a dirty public-house
existence ; the brutes are fed till one has the
distinction of mating with a queen and then all
are ruthlessly slaughtered.

Here is a community which has worked out
its problem. Does the same fate await mankind ?
We have seen that the psychology of unconscious
woman, of the flapper, has much in common
with that of the bee. As economic conditions
become more stringent, has the male much
chance ? Women are becoming emancipated,
bigger and stronger in body and brain ; the best
of them are overtopping men. The inferiority of
women as citizens is becoming less marked.
When they can do all that a man can do, while
at the same time having the power to carry on
the race, what will happen when restriction of
population becomes a dire necessity ?

We have a tendency to revert to our origins ;
we begin and end as long-heads. The female was
the first and she may be the last. But as the
last long-head is different from the first, so is the

last female. If the short-head has been devoured, absorbed, his qualities have been absorbed with him ; if the male is created for the purposes of the female, he was so created that she might acquire his qualities, and that the race might benefit by the cleavage. In the same way the unconscious may be the eternal, but the last unconscious will be different from the first, and this through the creation of the conscious. We shall consider this later with Geley, for conscious and unconscious are the greatest of the dualities, and if we can solve their problem we solve the problem of evolution.

Woman the unconscious becomes more and more imbued with consciousness ; she does not lose her unconscious birthright, but it is transmuted.

Woman, the emotional, the instinctive, the eternal, the materialist, is obviously a representative of the unconscious ; man, experimenting, specializing, co-ordinating, planning, individual in his activities, idealizing, abstracting, is the exponent of the conscious qualities.

Woman, conservative yet looking to the future, sensuous, intuitive, ancient yet abiding, absorbent, imaginative, creative, is the prototype of the Mediterranean or Eurafrican or Hamitic

Race; man, with his strength, his will, his egotism, his logic, his intellect, represents the Asiatic.

The Roman Law throbs with maleness, and it is the code of the Asiatics. Where Roman and patriarchal principles dominate, the male is always supreme. Woman's position in Rome, in Sparta, in Prussia, was an unenviable one. Yet the Mediterranean women did not surrender without a struggle. Women unconsciously control the race, and probably suffered this domination for their own good; *elles reculaient pour mieux sauter.* On the fringes of the Empire, notably in Asia Minor, they held to their old ideas of mother-right, and gradually came to hold magistracies. In France and Italy they were repressed and are to some extent to-day, but they are still strong in unconscious femininity; though woman in France to-day is not so politically emancipated as her English sister, she has governed Europe from her *salons.* Individually she is more sure of herself, more natural, than the Englishwoman. She is the controlling partner in marriage. One of the wise observations of Dr. Emil Reich was that the French woman was as superior to the French man as the English man was to the English woman.

That is to say, the Mediterranean women have in a way always retained their superiority. The French woman does not, like her English sister, suffer from mental conflicts. If you make an assignation with an Englishwoman she does not keep it; her unconscious accepts, her conscious thinks better of it. A Frenchwoman keeps her appointments; why should she not? She is a queen and has always been one. I will illustrate my remarks by a newspaper cutting from Mrs. Patrick Campbell's *Life and Letters* in the *Queen*. She is talking of Sarah Bernhardt.

" I remember one night a discussion we had on ' flirting.' Sarah took this word very seriously; she said that flirting stirred and excited animal passion. That flirting was a peculiarity of English men and women."

" A Frenchwoman loves and gives herself; but to excite passion *pour passer le temps*—' never,' she declared."

An Englishwoman feels her unconscious and dares no more than play with it; there is a continual conflict within her between unconscious and conscious. The true ideal is Geley's, the unconscious thoroughly imbued with consciousness.

We have noted the high position held by

women in Ancient Egypt and in Ireland. The Mediterranean Race meant woman triumphant. The strange thing is that the ancients, in their unconsciousness, seemed to have themselves recognized the essential maleness and femaleness of the races.

I have mentioned the Hittite sculpture of Iasily Kaya depicting the meeting of male and female gods for fertility. An interesting instance has recently been given by Mr. W. J. Perry in *The Megalithic Culture of Indonesia*. Menhirs are associated with men, and table stones with women. To ensure the stability of a village it is necessary to have a male and female stone set side by side—a dissolith. We have glimpses there of a sky people and an earth people—as we might say, a Jupiter people and a Gē people. Unconsciously the principle of race-marriage seems to have been recognized even in ancient times. A neolithic object recently found in Malta has been described by Professor Zammit in *The Hal-Tarxien Neolithic Temple, Malta* (Oxford, 1916). It appears to represent two phalli standing on a pitted base and the whole seems to have been enclosed by a dolmen. The phalli represent the male principle, and the pitted base the female. There is a more potent sign than duality and that is trinity of finality, and that appears to be symbolized in Malta by the dolmen, two upright stones and one transom ; it seems to typify nature working through duality to a higher unity, a unity in trinity. We seem now to be in a better position to answer the question of my friend, the padre ; what is the object of the struggle, and is it to continue eternally. Strife is merged in love ; the cleavage was for the higher development of humanity ; and the solution of differences gives a higher unity.

CHAPTER IX

CONSCIOUS AND UNCONSCIOUS.

A new significance attaches to the terms *conscious* and *unconscious* owing to the work of Freud and his disciples. It would be outside the scope of this volume to delve into the matter too deeply, but we have used the expressions in regard to race psychology and I want to emphasize what the terms mean for us. In scientific research to-day, in the hopelessness of finding out what things are, we are content to consider more and more what they do. Probably we can never know the essential nature of things, and to try to do so may be a waste of time. Gradually we are coming to adopt the more simple and practical point of view that the nature of a thing lies in what it does. We cannot say what electricity is, but we learn more and more as to its functions. Sir Oliver Lodge's complicated mechanisms are discredited, and we associate electricity more and more with action, even that once unspeakable thing, action at a distance. "Action," says Professor Eddington in *Space Time and Gravitation*, " is generally regarded as the most fundamental thing in the real work of physics," and we work accordingly with our new units of action, bringing in the element of time so significant in Bergsonian philosophy. And so with the mind ; less and less are we able to find out what it is, but more and more do we find out what it does. We are becoming more inductive and less deductive, as our Mediterraneanism increases. In this volume we have taken a wide survey of what the mind does, wider than is the practice with most psychologists, who deal more or less with a normal, abstract mind. If we are to define the mind in terms of action, our racial investigations should afford us a wider standpoint, and it is not to be wondered at if our conceptions of conscious and unconscious take on a new colouring from our wider experience.

The instigator, if not the founder, of the New Psychology, is Freud, a Viennese practitioner, who, in his dealings with neuropaths found that most of their troubles arose from the workings of the unconscious. We live ordinarily in a conscious life, aware of our wishes, our impressions and our actions. The neuropath acts in an abnormal manner, as if not thoroughly controlled by conscious will and morality. Such phenomena were found by Freud to be generally due to some unconscious wish being thwarted, some catastrophe in the unconscious life. Such wishes and desires are then thrust down into the unconscious and repressed, where they retaliate by forming complexes which seem to possess little personalities of their own, like Miss Beauchamp's, constantly at war with the main personality and often overthrowing it. One of the great manifestations of the unconscious is the dream, and therein our unconscious wishes fulfil themselves in so far as they are permitted to do so by the *censor* of our morality. In order to find out the cause of these cataclysms Freud tapped the unconscious life ; he got his patients to tell him their dreams, of which he is the first great interpreter ; and he put them into a semi-comatose state and let them speak at random from their unconscious unfettered by conscious control. Sometimes he discovered the secret of their unconscious by their actions, for he has discovered that accident plays a far less important part in these than we had supposed. In an amusing work, *The Psychopathology of Every-*

day Life, he shews that what we do purposely
are our conscious actions, but what we do
accidentally are often the actions of our
unconscious wishes. From the results of these
observations Freud was generally able to identify
the unconscious complex at the root of the
trouble, and, strangely enough, when the
complex was thus isolated and explained to the
patient it was solved and the patient was cured.
It seems that in recognizing and understanding
his complex the patient asserted the domination
of his conscious over it, and he became properly
capped again.

Freud's work was taken up and developed by
his brilliant disciple Jung, who has carried his
master's principles into ethnology; what the
dream is to the individual, the myth is to the
race. And so we have our racial complexes and
racial methods of solving them. We cannot help
having observed some of these in our consideration of the races, and later we may consider
others. A general review of the Freudian work
will be found in Mr. Wilfrid Lay's *Man's Unconscious Conflict*, an exceedingly useful summary,
marred by that prejudice in favour of morality
and the conscious which at present dominates
the American people.

The prejudice against Freud and his unconscious is somewhat general ; his unconscious is
nearly always sexual, infantile, primitive, and
people have come to regard it individually as
something to be ashamed of. But it must be
remembered that Freud was first and foremost
a practitioner. He saw the disease and set
himself to cure it. It was not his fault if the
disease was the infantile unconscious. The
mistake has been to call this pathological
unconscious *the* unconscious. There is a great
unconscious and a small one ; a normal and a
pathological one. The unconscious when repressed reverts to infantilism and barbarity, but
this is only owing to unnatural repression.
The later Freudians have seen in the unconscious,
the *libido*, the life force. If ordinarily it exhibits
itself in a threefold manifestation as a desire to
eat, a desire to work, and a desire to reproduce,
it is still argued that the three manifestations
are essentially of one thing. Sex, as we have
seen, arose from the act of devouring ; and when
man, in a growing civilization, found his sexual
appetites repressed, he prodded in the earth and
invented agriculture ; rubbed sticks together
and made fire ; sighing for his lost mistress he
explored the country and discovered art and

æsthetics. It is for this reason that man, rather than woman, has become a technician, an artist and a specialist. His activities arose from a repression which woman never suffered in the same degree, for woman's sexuality has not the explosive character of the male.

We thus reach a broader view of the *libido*, the life force, of which we have seen that woman and the Mediterraneans are so full.

But as if to prove that the unconscious mind does not work independently but has a subterranean unity, we find these ideas being worked out elsewhere, particularly in France and Belgium, independently of Freud. Bergson, Maeterlinck, Geley, Montessori, are only further instances of the neo-Hamitism; in different words and images they express the same thing.

2

Maeterlinck seems to overestimate the conscious—at least in *Wisdom and Destiny*. He thinks that those armed with wisdom can stand unshaken before the blows of fate. I admit that his Wisdom is not entirely the conscious, for with him reason is the conscious, and he acknowledges its insufficiency. Reason is a negative thing; but wisdom is positive. The unconscious is the enemy, as with the Freudians.

" In unconsciousness we ever must dwell, but
are able to purify, day after day, the unconsciousness that wraps us around." But there is very
much more in Maeterlinck than this ; we find
thoughts so profound as : " Nothing befalls us
that is not of the nature of ourselves," a saying
which is really prophetic of the theory of
relativity. Everything has its natural path.
We too have our natural paths, our own paths ;
If Winter Comes has this for its theme. " None
but yourself shall you meet in the highway of
fate."

Like most inspired writers, Maeterlinck is
greater than himself. He hangs prophesies in
the air, without support, and yet we cannot but
realize their truth. His ideas are greater than
his reasoning. *The Life of the Bee* is full of these
deep, mysterious sayings ; and they are all
prophetic. They find their scientific basis in
Geley and Rutherford.

He tells us how Reaumur put a mathematical
problem to Koenig—given certain materials and
conditions, to work out mathematically the most
economical system of containers. Koenig arrived
at the cell of the honey-bee. Then Maeterlinck
holds up his hands in wonder that the bee should
have acted as if it had been a perfect mathe-

matician. The wonder is of quite a different character : it is that the mathematician should have proved as good as the bee.

His attitude is that the bee works so wonderfully that we must ascribe to it some unaccountable intelligence. Lower nature is unendowed with reason, and yet it moves. We have yet to realize that what can be done with intelligence can very often be done much better without it.

The conscious is a thing of late birth and doubtful antecedents. Puffed up with an upstart's arrogance she turns round on nature saying, " You exist solely through my perception; you are my creation." Nature can afford to laugh in her sleeve. She is really rather proud of this child of her old age, and treats it kindly ; she sees in it useful possibilities.

If Geley is the first to give us an adequate explanation of the purpose of the conscious, I feel that Maeterlinck has more than an inkling of it. Although he definitely belittles the unconscious, yet in a broader, more indefinite way, he magnifies it. What is *The Betrothal* but an epic of the unconscious ? The ancestors, right back to the Great Ancestor, possibly the pithecanthropus, take a hand in choosing Tyltyl's mate ; but not only the ancestors, the unborn also; in fact they are more insistent. What is this but the recognition of an unconscious stretching back and fore illimitably into past and future?

Nor is he without a definite feeling as to how the unconscious works. Of Nature, he says in *The Life of the Bee*, " she appears to be constantly blundering, no less in the world of her first experiments than in that of her last, man." But she has her very definite tools : " the idea, however, has now grown aware of its strength "; and again : " It is certain that whenever the infinite mass allows us to seize the appearance of an idea, the appearance takes this road whereof we know not the end." Nature progresses through the idea.

And this brings us again to *Wisdom and Destiny*, reason negative, wisdom positive ; and the soul compounded of wisdom. What is the other component ? Possibly imagination or the idea. On the whole Maeterlinck leads easily to Geley, for he shews us unconscious nature, experimenting, sometimes blundering, working through the idea, finally evolving the conscious.

3

Maeterlinck's wisdom is a much higher thing than reason, for it possesses a certain freedom and an emotional support. He does not seem to make it clear what is the distinction between the two. For that we want a more scientific treatment, such as we find in *The Freudian Wish* by Mr. Holt.

There is no glorificatoin of the reason here. Man simply behaves. His behaviour is a function of his environment. His responses to external stimuli have become integrated in character. He responds as a whole to the external world, and his response is his behaviour, his character. Hamlet's Horatio was a properly integrated man —a man you could rely on ; you knew what he would do in certain circumstances. His antipodes is Hamlet himself, the failure, suffering from thwarted integration, a Freudian neurotic. The good man is fully integrated and free ; the bad man is badly integrated and a slave. The former carries out his wish, with the latter the wish is thwarted.

I think Mr. Holt leaves out a small step in his reasoning. Let us consider the unregenerate Undine or Arthur Payne in *The Tragic Bride*. They repress no wish ; they are free ; but both are sinners, acting anti-socially. As Mr. Holt clearly shews, the only salvation is knowledge ; he says that all the more embracing behaviour formulæ are moral. That is, to be moral, they must be embracing. In the breath of knowledge and wisdom we shall act morally. This is the keynote of Socrates' teaching and really of Christ's. " Father, forgive them, for they know not what they do." Wisdom, virtue and freedom are synonymous terms.

But if to be wise is to be good, what becomes of behaviourism, of natural reaction to environment ? The answer contains the crux of the matter. There are two kinds of environment, the real and the ideal. Responding naturally to real environment we avoid mental conflict and are moral individually. Reacting to the ideal environment we are socially moral.

This is where the importance of wisdom is manifest. We can only wish the right thing by knowing, by being wise. The environment is thus enlarged by an ideal content. We still respond to the environment, but it is a bigger environment.

Here, I think, is a great function of the conscious. Holt thinks it merely registers the response to the environment, but it does more than that. In registering responses it builds up the ideal content, it provides an ideal world. This is what Maeterlinck is driving at. The conscious helps to build up wisdom and what Maeterlinck calls the soul. The young Undine and Arthur Payne were natural sinners; they had no souls.

The point is very important racially. Brigadier Gerard scandalized the hunting-field by killing the fox with his sword. He responded quite naturally to his environment: there was the fox to be killed and he killed it. The English hunting men, however, were under the ban of the ideal content; the fox had to be killed in a certain way. That is the spirit of all sport: you have to do a thing in a certain prescribed manner. There are rules to every game, and they are the ideal content. This kind of idealism, strong in the English, and, in a varying way, in the Teutons generally, is weak in the Latin races. The materialists of Europe were the French and Italians, and are now the French, and the trait is visible not only in games but in the matter of reparations, indemnities and the treatment of a fallen foe.

The question has been recently further elucidated by Dr. Brown in *Psychology and Psychotherapy*, a valuable book not only in that it does so much to confirm Freud's theories as applied to practical work among those suffering from shell-shock and the various shattering experiences of war, but more particularly in its reference to Bergson's *Matter and Memory*. Bergson falls into line with the actionists. Our body is an instrument of action and action solely ; our brain is merely a motor organ. He is in line with Holt in saying that we merely re-act ; but if we re-act through the brain there is a certain freedom. Perception is merely an act of selection, a selection of the method of acting. Things are what they seem, they are not fictions of the idealist's brain. This is perhaps clearly brought out by an example in Mr. Pycraft's *Courtship of Animals* : if a spider on a leaf simulates the excrement of a bird, we may feel convinced that such an object appears to us just as it does to the bird. But if things are as they appear, we only see part of them ; we see them in the light of our virtual action upon them, and space is a relation of objects to such action.

But when he comes to memory Bergson sees something quite different. Memory is spirit. He speaks of pure memory, a virtual state, which passes into actual perception. We thus get an idea not of perception passing into memory but of memory as a pure and absolute thing emerging into perception.

The conception very much resembles Holt's ; we have less mechanism, more relativity. In the days when we spoke of inorganic matter we constructed elaborate theoretical machines to bring it into harmony with nature ; Sir Oliver Lodge constructs such machines in the ether. Since the birth of relativity we see that one object, one fact, bears relation to some other. We content ourselves with exploring the relation, which is the real bond between them.

It may seem confusing to have so many views of the working of the mind : Maeterlinck with his soul and wisdom, Holt with his behaviourism and knowledge, Bergson with his action and pure memory. But they are only aspects of the same thing. It is perhaps best to visualize these conceptions ; if we do not know what the mind is, let us be clear as to what it does, and if I too construct an artificial machine, let it be remembered that it is only an illustration of action. Let us imagine a simple spherical machine like a tank, having only one opening to the outside world. Through this and this alone the commander within can formulate his action ; through it he is aware of things and acts accordingly. This hole is not covered with glass but with a transparent photographic film which moves continuously past the aperture and is wound up on a spool. Though the commander could, by looking through the aperture, gain sufficient knowledge of his surroundings to act with reasonable success, he could hardly by this means plan out a campaign. Appearances are deceptive, darkness and distance lead to uncertainty, some things are totally unrecognizable. But the commander always has his spool to work on. In the night-time he can take it down, compare past with present, classify, theorize, make new plans in accordance with the record. Such a spool in the hands of a wise commander might well be called the soul of the tank. Looking through the hole is perception; the spool is memory; the activities connected with the spool are the ideal content, and the soul.

Mediterranean man had a large aperture and neglected the spool. Asiatic man had a poor aperture and neglected it. He thought only of the spool, and in time made a new spool of his own. Working on this he neglected his tank and the world outside, and thought that the spool was the world, and the creator thereof. He became a metaphysician.

Apparently what nature wanted was both the hole and the spool to be used in their fulness, the one correcting and amplifying the other.

It is in this way that we have regarded the races as conscious and unconscious, but the Freudians with their unconscious action and unconscious memory have complicated both the question and the tank. To meet them we must suppose that our commander came to realize in course of time that his tank was not what he had supposed it to be. He found that what he thought was the bottom of the tank was only a platform or deck, down through which the spool continued with its winding. As he examined his tank more and more closely he found that it was really in the nature of our bubble floating on a magma. He thought he had been steering his vessel, but now he realized that his vessel was often steering him. The magma had currents and it was open to him to follow them or to struggle against them; the latter course often met with disastrous consequences. The wise commander, having studied the theory of relativity, found it best to utilize his upper deck knowledge and experience in overcoming accidental deviations, and falling in with the natural track of the vessel along the main current.

We have already compared our races to such bubbles; the Asiatic is less deeply imbedded in the magna than the Mediterranean. With the first the deck is lower and the tank more of a complete sphere; with the second the deck is higher and the sphere less complete. The first has better developed hemispheres, a greater conscious loop; the second is less developed in this respect. The magma is the great unconscious, the general and ultimate life force, and the Mediterranean is deeply imbedded therein.

CHAPTER X

HOW NATURE WORKS.

It seems to me that a new era in evolution and philosophy is opened by Geley in *From the Unconscious to the Conscious*, but it was disappointing to find that the translation of his work into English met with the unconsidered suspicion of those who merely react.

Geley's work is partly philosophic and partly experimental. He follows Bergson in pointing out the inadequacy of the present theories of evolution. " Survival of the fittest " does not explain how a reptile which developed wings can survive. By developing or modifying a limb an animal generally becomes not more but less fit. " Adaptation to environment " does not help in a case where the environment is changed ; a fish by adapting itself to its environment renders itself less fit for life in the air, so that these two principles are not only negative but destructive as regards evolution.

The lives of the Sitaris and the hunting hymenoptera suggest that these creatures behave as if they had thought out their life history and the history of their young. It is as with the bee which behaves as if it were the most skilled mathematician. The conclusion is that there is something else which behaves just like intellect. Bergson calls it instinct; Geley has another name for it, but it is only a matter of terminology.

Then we have the case of the caterpillar dissolving itself into an almost amorphous quantity of matter in the chrysalis before developing into a butterfly. How can this dissolution and reconstruction take place without some plan and purpose working behind the mechanism? The current theories of evolution are purely mechanical and negative, mere schemes, and utterly unable to account for the dynamic and planning force behind the phenomena. There is a *diathesis* under which an animal is born with horns and cloven hoofs, or with wings, feathers and a beak. We know that a crustacean will repair a broken claw, and that a broken crystal will rebuild itself in its appropriate shape. There is a planning force behind it all, and this Geley calls a directing dynamo-psychism. Geley's conclusions are largely based

on his experiments with the medium Eva.
When hypnotized she produced from the orifices
of her body a film of what Dr. Geley considers
to be elemental matter, and out of this developed,
while Eva passed through pains as of labour,
hands and limbs and a beautiful face. This is
an act of birth, an act of creation, an act of the
unconscious.

In this connection some of the authenticated
examples of birth-marks, given by Mr. Heape in
Sex Antagonism, are of interest.

A lizard dropped from the ceiling upon the
naked breast of a pregnant woman. She was
badly frightened and declared that her child
would be born with a mark of a lizard on its
breast. The child was born with this mark.

A pregnant woman had a strong desire for
raspberries, and her child was born with the
mark of a raspberry upon its body.

A woman's fiancé returned from the war with
his face slashed in a cross, and her first child
was born with a similar slash.

A child was born with an amputated arm and
the marks of stitches on it. It was an illegiti-
mate child, and the arm was a replica of the
father's.

These are, as it were, negative instances.

For the positive Mr. Heape speaks with admiration of the wonderful corpus of practical knowledge possessed by breeders. Jacob was able
to influence the marking of his lambs by placing
peeled rods in view of the ewes. A breeder of
black cattle paints all his gates black. A
horse-breeder found that so long as he had his
mares covered in the dark the foals took after
the dam ; on his changing his tactics and allowing
the mares to look well at the sire, the foals took
after the sire.

It appears that the female, as a creative
machine or agent, is influenced by vision and
imitation. But the matter appears to go deeper
than that.

In *Suggestion and Auto-Suggestion* M. Baudouin
described the almost miraculous cures of M. Coué
and the New Nancy School, and we have since
had the opportunity of becoming acquainted
with the method through M. Coué's recent
lectures in London. The cures are indeed
effected by hypnotism, but the writer points out
that this is in reality self-hypnotism. It appears
that we have almost complete power over ourselves through imagination. It is the thought,
the imagination, which is creative ; the will is
in these matters negative. Fear, on the other

hand, is not merely negative, but in effect destructive imagination. It appears to account for the first series of Mr. Heape's examples of birth-marks.

It is interesting to quote again from Maeterlinck's *Life of the Bee.* Dealing with the evolution of the humble-bee, he says, " The idea, however, has now grown aware of its strength " ; and " it is certain that wherever the infinite mass allows us to seize the appearance of an idea, the appearance takes this road whereof we know not the end." That is, Nature appears to work through imagination or the idea.

As regards the negative or destructive part played by the will in these matters, we are reminded again of our two races, the one imaginative and the other the embodiment of the will. The latter seem to get what they want, but when they get it, they find they do not really want it, or that it is the wrong thing. A classic instance is perhaps Soames Forsyte breaking through every obstacle to get a son, and being presented with a daughter.

Geley does not emphasize the imagination. He points to nature striving, experimenting, trying to do something. Sometimes she succeeds, but evolution is strewn with her failures, scrapped machines. Of nature Maeterlinck says in *The Life of the Bee*: "She appears to be constantly blundering, no less in the world of her first experiments than in that of the last, of man."

What, according to Geley, is Nature, the great unconscious, trying to do? She is trying to become conscious. The unconscious becomes conscious in man, the representative in life of this great unconscious of Nature. We are constantly flooding the unconscious with unconsciousness. Having done our part in this work, we die and are taken back into the unconscious.

Success and happiness are satisfactory from the point of view of the conscious, but for the unconscious they are less effective than pain, unhappiness, and failure. For the latter give more experience, they do more of the work of flooding the unconscious with consciousness. We begin to gain some light on the problem of death, pain and failure. We begin to see more significance in the attitude of *Rabbi Ben Ezra*:

> " All, I could never be,
> All, men ignored in me,
> That I was worth to God whose
> wheel the pitcher shaped."

By this great unconscious behind our lives Geley would explain telepathy, mediumism, multiple personality, script writing, spiritual appearances. In our races we have seen that one is better, the other worse capped.

Whatever be the scientific basis for this theory of Geley's we have its counterpart in the great philosophies of life, Vedantism, Christianity and the philosophy of Schopenhauer : the Absolute and Eternal running on in a straight line ; life, appearance, the conscious, the will, breaking off and running parallel. But in these philosophies the new line proves to be a hopeless mistake ; the only solution is to put an end to life, to destroy it and drop again into nirvana, the. eternal.

Geley is more hopeful. He thinks the conscious life has some purpose. The unconscious, striving to become conscious of itself, has deliberately created it, and the end is the permeating of the unconscious by the conscious.

2

In the scientific sense it is perhaps a little difficult to place this unconscious which is trying to do something, trying to make itself conscious. An elemental unconscious force could not know of the conscious, much less try to become it. When we survey Geley's evolution strewn with scrapped experiments, when we consider the hypertrophied ornaments described in Mr. Pycraft's *Courtship of Animals*, we are much more inclined to think of a conscious developing by accident, and kept, like the male, because it was useful.

But we know so little, and this new unconscious is so wonderful in its secret ways that we must not dogmatize. It appears from M. Coué's work that the human imagination is definitely creative. If it should eventuate that the creative force *is* thought and imagination it would not now be surprising.

Yet probably our thoughts are confined to things of which we become aware through the experience : our thoughts seem to be imitative. And even if our imagination be inspired by an idea outside our experience, we have possibly a fund of knowledge in the great unconscious with its universal memory, so that thought again reflects experience. We see here, however, the significance of the accident and the sport. If one generation or one experience were the exact replica of another, our thoughts would be stunted in their growth and there could be little progress ; an accidental occurrence or juxtaposition or growth may be not only useful in itself but may give birth to an idea, altering the whole course of evolution. And herein we find a special significance attaching to the male, the experimenter, and the short-head, the idealist.

Our workaday view of nature would be that she is trying to do something; she has an urge, but towards what she knows not. Things happen, and she perpetuates the happenings that suit her. Dr. Geley throws cold water on Bergson's comparison of evolution to a sheaf of rockets with God at its centre; of intelligence to the ascending energy of the fireworks and matter to the dead sticks falling back to earth.

But does not this metaphor really present the most helpful view of the case? We have considered two parallel developments, the two races and sex. In both these cases we have strife and opposition. We see in a way that love is strife and strife is love. Is not, in the same way, the conscious at once the enemy and complement of the conscious; her child who is at once her enemy and her lover; is not their difference finally solved in the blending of marriage?

It seems to me that in some such turning round on herself as Bergson supposes in the image of the rockets the unconscious becomes conscious. It is only in opposition that a force can become aware of itself, realize itself. And

M

this, it seems from Geley, is just what the unconscious is striving to do.

A single elemental force would be represented graphically by a straight line or a set of parallel straight lines. This is " the natural path." Let some slight accident intervene and the force turns on itself and a whirl is set up.

Has experimental science any place for this elemental and eternal unconscious of Geley? It is curious that Geley's work should appear at the same time as Prof. Rutherford's publication of his work on electricity and matter. Matter is but a whirl of electricity, negative electrons, revolving around a positive nucleus. The nucleus is the balance to the negative electron. " Hence, in the ultimate," says Prof. Rutherford, " matter disappears and electricity alone remains."

If we are to find some scientific basis for the unconscious, it must be something ultimate, and the ultimate thing for natural science is negative electricity. Has this any connection with the unconscious? As far as we know they both seem ultimate things, and may ultimately be the same thing. We know that women, representatives of the unconscious, are very full of electricity. Popular parlance, which often has an inkling of the truth, speaks of the unconscious power of certain individuals as personal magnetism.

Such a theory would explain many things : how a woman polarizes a man ; how attraction between the sexes gives rise to repulsion ; the horror of incest would be an instance of electrical repulsion.

But until we know more about both terms of the comparison it is not safe to be definite. Yet note the similarity of the courses of development. In evolution we have first electricity which becomes matter, living matter, the conscious. In psychology we have first the unconscious from which in turn arise matter, living matter, the conscious. The origins of the same things cannot well be different, and if our reasoning is correct the unconscious may ultimately be found to be electricity. We know far more than we realize, and it is interesting to note that Miss Marie Corelli arrived at a similar conclusion in *The Romance of Two Worlds*.

CHAPTER XI

THE CONSCIOUS

Nature seems to have hit on the conscious accidentally, as a means of realizing herself. Through an accidental swerve the life force turned round upon itself, realizing itself in reaction and opposition. In two special ways nature seems to have achieved the growth of the conscious, in the male and in the short-headed race ; and both ways were accidental. Starvation led to cannabilism, which in time developed into sex mating. Isolation in the mountains appears to have given rise to cretinism and the Mongol.

As this volume is mainly concerned with race it is necessary to consider more precisely how the brachycephal represents the conscious principle. The mentality of both races is compounded of both conscious and unconscious elements ; but with the short-heads the conscious preponderates. A study of the pathological mongol, well known

to our practitioners, shews that in this aberrant
and defective type we have not only the somatic
characters of the Mongolian people, but also an
aberrant type of mind, referred to as mongol
idiocy. The patient suffers from what is popularly known as swelled-head. An aberrant type
of mind implies a mind which breaks away from
tradition and thereby asserts a kind of independence. This feature, once established, becomes
emphasized and in time we get the mind which
lives in the ideal rather than the real, creating a
world of its own. We get the idealist and the
metaphysician ; a personality which not merely
re-acts, but considers, schemes and co-ordinates.
In a primitive society such men were looked up to
with considerable respect, for they could not only
remember, they could make use of their memory.
They could make cunning plans for the defeat
of neighbouring tribes. Of such a kind were
Ulysses and Ensor Doone ; among the Mongolians
such men were regarded with awe.

It has been remarked that all deviations from
the normal type are pathological ; from such an
accidental and pathological circumstance appears
to arise the conscious mind, and its resulting
independence and freedom. Being found useful,
it was perpetuated. The short head meant the

high head, with well-developed hemispheres ; and from its shape arose a power of co-ordination which seems to arise from its physical construction. In its more pathological aspects it idealizes to excess ; becoming normalized it registers, coordinates, directs.

2

When we find such an acute thinker as Mr. Bertrand Russell telling us that most of our logic and philosophy are wrong ; when we discover that the intelligence of the world has been traversing a blind alley for the last two thousand years ; when we perceive our state machinery so clogged with grey matter that action is well nigh impossible ; when we see the results of intellectualism, idealism and system in Germany ; we may well be excused in wondering whether the conscious is not a mistake.

Has the conscious a useful function, and if so, what ? I mean, humanly speaking, quite apart from the broader issues of the last chapter. If we desire to discover an example of the proper working of the conscious, I think we find it in the Romans. Before them the world was characterless and chaotic. The Romans invented and perpetuated system, law and order. Out of the varying external they evolved an ideal unified code, a code, which would meet all conditions. And the Roman system had a definite object— orderly social life, Aristotle's "good life." There was no vague and purposeless idea of Rome's supremacy; no sheer power or sheer intelligence; no pure reason or categorical imperative. The Romans were neither tyrants nor metaphysicians. There was no idea of power for the sake of power. It was power to an end.

And that is the proper working of the conscious.

Imagine a path which crosses a ravine. The savage scrambles down one side and up the other. Not very difficult, not very inconvenient in simple circumstances. But taking time, awkward on occasion. The white man comes and builds a bridge. The savage laughs to see the expenditure of time and energy on this mere crossing of the cañon. But when the work is done, it is much easier and quicker for everyone; and you can do things which you could not before; you can take a car-load of passengers over at a time. That is the true function of the conscious; a system, a labour-saving device, a machine. Or if you regard the unconscious as a reservoir, the conscious is the regulative tap.

Logic, mathematics are such machines. In

Our Knowledge of the External World Mr.
Bertrand Russell finds the classical philosophy,
logic and metaphysics pathological. We might
suspect something of the sort since they are the
products of a pathological cranium. He tells us
that the Hegelism of *Appearance and Reality* is
built up on bad logic, the classic logic which only
recognises subject and predicate ; which did not
recognise relations ;   which, in its egotism,
recognised nothing outside itself. And so the
old geometry falls before *Relativity* which recognises that everything has its own path, not the
egotistic path of the thinker.

But even Mr. Russell cannot entirely escape
from Asiaticism. He says that some knowledge
is general and primitive, and gives the following
proposition as an example : " If anything has a
certain property, and whatever has this property
has a certain other property, then the thing in
question has this other property." Particularis-
ing he gives the following example, which he
says is formally true : " If Socrates is a man, and
all men are mortal, then Socrates is mortal."

These do not appear to be knowledge but
dummy machines. The real working machine
is his other example, which he excludes from
pure logic : " Socrates is a man, all men are

mortal, therefore Socrates is mortal." This is a
slot-machine, and the words " all men are mortal,
therefore" constitute the works. " Man " is
the slot, " mortal" is the ticket. Put in the
coin " Socrates " or " Lloyd George," and you
get your ticket, " mortal." " Mount Vesuvius "
does not fit the slot, or is returned. If the
machine is badly constructed, instead of a ticket
you are apt to get cigarettes or a bottle of scent.
Mathematical formulæ are machines of the same
kind.

The mistake is to think that logic and mathematics are more than machines, or to imagine
that you can get out of them or out of philosophy
more than you put into them. Mathematics,
logic, are formulæ, time-savers. Instead of each
man traversing the cañon, all can go across in
a car. The only way to increase knowledge is to
increase experience ; the other things are mere
aids. If all the time given to metaphysics had
been devoted to natural science, we should be in
a very different position now. Look at our
philosophy to-day, barren, useless, maundering
pathologically round the ruins of Aristotle and
Kant ; follow Professor Rutherford into the
laboratory and see the absolute and definite
origin of matter.

Some people build bridges where there is no
chasm : they are the metaphysicians. Some
multiply bridges, and the public pays.

But possibly in another way there is a kind of
general absolute knowledge. If there is anything in the story of the Pentecost, this must be
so—a knowledge transcending personal experience. Personally I feel convinced of it,
mainly on Freudian grounds. My personal
experience leads me to believe that the Freudian
dream-symbolism is correct, namely, that in
dreams certain ideas take certain definite shapes,
like baskets, hats and shoes. With all persons
they appear to take these shapes. And the
success of the psycho-analysts is largely based on
this catholic representation. Other examples
are the British bull-dog and Mr. Horrabin's
Japhet. This seems to me to indicate a kind of
absolute knowledge, apart from experience.

What the dream is to the individual, mythology
is to the race, and superstition to mankind. In
mythology a certain track is laid down for the
hero ; his natural path is the track of the sun.
He is virgin-born, he is swallowed by Mother-
earth, he rises again ; he is immortal. Into
this scheme fall Jesus Christ, Jonah, King
Arthur, the Wandering Jew. Lord Kitchener is

not allowed to die. The tradition is not without some historical colour afforded by such examples as William the Conqueror and Erasmus. Forty years ago the water-diviner was scoffed at by the educated, but to-day, ceasing from our attempts to construct the mechanism, we are content to recognize that he has some relation to water; and possibly we should not necessarily condemn astrology and palmistry because we fail to discover connecting links. Chevreul's pendulum has for centuries been used in divination. It is now used practically by M. Coué as a psychological machine, and generally as a sexometer. It is also, I believe, a race-indicator; as far as my experience goes, it does not work for the short-heads. As a sex indicator it seems to adopt the symbolism of the phallus and the lingam.

Another matter in which we are shewing more sympathy is our treatment of children. Now that we have ceased to dragoon them, they begin to astonish us by their genius, their insight, their intuitive grasp. Our methods are no longer those of a crammer, and our teaching seems more and more to be merely an awakening of knowledge that is already there. Is it possible that we really know everything, merely failing in realization ?

It is said that when a savage first sees a battleship he is not surprised, he simply cannot realize it. While man's sexual appetites were satisfied it is supposed that he did not realize nature. I really think that is our general attitude : we are more or less aware of external things, but we do not realize them until for some reason the interest is awakened. Possibly what we call knowledge is in effect such realization.

In the light of the new psychology such absolute knowledge is not at all impossible. If beneath us stretches the one great unconscious, unbounded in space or time, such a conception would be quite comprehensible.

CHAPTER XII

CONCLUSIONS

As living matter becomes divided into male and female, for the purposes of higher development ; that the female may be fructified by the male ; that he may experiment and specialize and that she may reap the fruit for the race ; as their relations are of strife which is resolved in love ; so, reverting to our races, we find an emotional, naturalistic, dynamic, creative, characterless, fickle, undependable people brought into contact with and ultimately dominated by a race whose characters are bravery, force, system, co-ordination, intellect, idealism and will. Here too strife leads to marraige, and ultimately to the extinction externally of the dominant partner. Unless the older race has in its experiences managed to absorb and acquire the qualities of the newer, this experiment of nature has been in vain.

When the race marriage is perfect we have

those periods of efflorescence which gave us the art and literature of Periclean Athens, or the literature and political success of Elizabethan England. Taine thinks that such flourishing periods in letters correspond to a developed power in the nation, *une puissance dévéloppée ;* in the light of our arguments we might venture to call them honeymoons.

Some ascribe the fall of Greece and Rome to intermarriage of the patrician classes ; it is probably safer to ascribe it to the absorbent powers of the long-heads. The tragedy of Greece and Rome is that the qualities of the Asiatics should have disappeared with the race who possessed them. The consideration has the greater importance in that it vitally affects ourselves. The disappearance of the short-heads has been accompanied by a long sweep of the pendulum in the direction of Hamitism. When we changed our allegiance and ranged ourselves alongside the Mediterraneans in the Great War we deliberately turned our backs on many of the qualities to which we owe our greatness.

Men like Adam Smith, Mill, Ricardo, practising theorists, are no longer a guide to our statesmen, and possibly many of our politicians could not understand them. The advent of the business man means action *ad hoc* ; our statesmen become opportunists. There is, to apply our metaphor of the tank, too much of the film and too little of the spool ; direct action without reference to the ideal content, memory, plan, system ; the universal gives way to the particular.

More obviously perhaps is this character manifested in journalism. If anything happens, the tendency is merely to react. The obvious is noticed, but what lies behind it is either not seen or is glossed over. Both good and bad actions are criticised, the bad because they are bad, the good because they are suspected to be hypocritical. In the more spacious days of Burke and Fox our countrymen seem to have looked a little beyond the obvious.

One of the characters of the more conscious mind is that its idealism embraces that which is not obvious. Its co-ordinating power, its recourse to memory, enable it to fill out the picture ; in a kind of higher sympathy it puts itself in the place of the object of criticism ; it views an action in its remoter bearings. Now we suffer from short-circuits ; our reactions do not pass through the loop of the hemispheres.

In journalism there is much mud-slinging with the hope that some of it may stick, too often an appeal to the envy, hatred and malice of the infantile unconscious. Our newspapers have but to raise the cry " Somebody must go " or " make them pay," and the infantile unconscious of the mob is immediately awakened. There is an absence of fairness, control, judgment, and a considerable falling off of intelligence. People will no longer read newspapers, they want to see pictures. For the same reason a good play has little chance against the attraction of the movies. If, before, the eye yielded place to the brain, now the brain is atrophied in the ascendancy of the eye.

The great harm in this growth of vision and reactionism is perhaps hardly sufficiently appreciated. We have a vague idea that the cinema is responsible for much moral obliquity, especially among children, but we are not sure how it happens. In this connexion we must think of the work of M. Coué, or the words of Maeterlinck : " It is certain that wherever the infinite mass allows us to seize the appearance of an idea, the appearance takes this road whereof we know not the end." When fortuitously nature created a mind which was capable of ideas, she accomplished a mechanism which was itself creative. In this way perhaps the characters of fiction are of more importance than those of real life. If a Soames Forsyte or a Mr. Pickwick ever existed their importance is trivial compared with the fictitious personages.

Imagination may be a part of Nature's creative force, yet the imagination must always be in some sense imitative. The boundlessness of the imagination forms the subject of one of Addison's essays; owing to its freedom from material fetters it may roam at will, almost without restrictions. And if its only limits be experience, whether in a narrower or a wider sense, yet its freedom allows such innumerable combinations that its creative power approaches the absolute.

Maeterlinck hints to us that any such ideal creation may be adapted into the evolutionary scheme. As in birthmarks, the ideal may become material. And no action or character of fiction passes without its creative result. Hence the representation of an act is the birth of an act itself; and an irresponsible statement in a newspaper has practical force from the moment it is printed.

When Tennyson said that more things are wrought by prayer than this world dreams of, he was perhaps anticipating Coué. The force of the prayer was in the imagination of its accomplishment. All prayers are effective in that they are creative, and no thought is conceived by the individual without its effect upon the community. Personal experience will convince everyone of this, and perhaps here we have an instance of that solidarity which binds us all together through the unconscious.

One of our great national assets is our freedom, not in its old sense, but regarded as a *penchant* for individuality. In no other country will you find such extremes, both of good and bad. And since the dice are loaded in favour of the good, we may take credit for an enormous volume of good thought, both personal and in fiction. Many modern novels are remarkable in this way, and probably at no time in the world's history was there such an output of good thought. We may almost say that as a nation thinks, so it is.

Mrs. Asquith has complained that our literature becomes more and more sexual, but that is probably all to the good. We have our national as well as our personal complexes. The great complex of the Greeks was *necessity*, a lesser one *incest*; ours, in the growing and often unnecessary restrictions of civilization, is

sex. Milton rose high above the prejudices of
his period when in the *Areopagitica* he pleaded
for the freedom of the press; perhaps like
Aristotle he knew that in this way a people
worked off its complexes in the play-attitude.
Literature is in this respect like our dreams. In
France sex can hardly be said to be repressed,
but with us it is, and it is women who feel more
and more the pinch of the shoe; and it is women
writers who most conspicuously work off their
complex in literature. In one of Mr. Hugh
Walpole's tales, a writer of the old school
passionately exclaims that he will be like the
moderns and call every part of the body by its
name. By calling a spade a spade we adopt the
Freudian method of psychotherapy, unveiling
and dissipating our complexes.

A very wholesome tendency is growing up of
laughing at our own faults, regarding ourselves
objectively. We are learning the wisdom of the
Greek " Know thyself." This, too, is Freudian.
The only way to resolve a complex is to diagnose
and know it. In *General Post* we laugh at the
idealism, the migratory ego of Sir Dennis
Broughton, who is not only a volunteer but in
his own imagination has always been one;
in Chapin's *New Morality*, at the numerous

screens of convention, really herd instinct, with which Colonel Jones hides his true feelings, while the women go straight for the essential business of the unconscious, tearing each other's hair.

One of our racial reversions is towards catholicism, another towards gambling; and gambling is as characteristic of the catholic and the Mediterranean as it is antagonistic to the Scot or the dissenter. It expresses a blind faith in Providence, otherwise the unconscious. Unfortunately we cannot all be in the special keeping of the eternal, but there is yet something of essential truth behind the gambling spirit. Just as some people are good card-holders, so others are successful gamblers. But my experience is that if it is in the natural path of some to back winners, to others it falls to back the second or the last horse.

While the Mediterranean, even in Cornwall, still hobbles his cattle, bringing rage to the heart of animal-lovers, the Asiatic drove his herds before him. He dealt in gross, and became in time a grocer, but in a wholesale way, like the Quakers; the Mediterraneans have always been hucksters. Houston Chamberlain remarks on the pococurantism of the Asiatic, his high *insouciance*, enabling him, in his idealism, to trust the man on the spot, and not to worry over trifles ; it was largely owing to the carping of the Market Place that Athens lost her superiority ; the pure reactionism of the Mediterranean often degenerates into the infantile. The Roman and British Empires are built up on pococurantism. The number and nature of our parliamentary questions to-day shews a Hamitic reversion.

And as regards individual life, what is to be our attitude in this strife between the conscious and the unconscious ? Are we to lie on the sea of chance and let it bear us whither it will ? Or are we to steer our individual course regardless of circumstances ? We have seen that the conscious is necessary as a tool, as a machine. Hypertrophied it leads us away from life, to inanity or disaster. By wisdom again, involving the conscious, we enlarge our environment by an ideal content. The more wise we are, the more morally we shall act. Thus we approach that true wisdom of Maeterlinck.

We have learnt that the will is often destructive, the thought creative. The first, inculcated by our taciturn forefathers, causes endless mental conflicts among their descendants, notably amongst women. One tries year after year to pass an examination, another thinks her salvation lies in practising music, another in bridge. Like determined golfers, the more they will the less they succeed. They are probably on the wrong track. If they had patience and submission their natural path might be revealed. " Nothing befalls us that is not of the nature of ourselves."

Even Maeterlinck in his wisdom seems to have left a blank. If our heads emerge into freedom, we are bound by the feet ; and if we have our natural paths, they must lie in the path of the great unconscious. We have not only to learn, but to wait and contemplate ; humbly, patiently to seek out what the eternal requires us to do, and do that.